Discover Complementary Healthcare

What is it? The easiest, simplest thing in the world - with it comes great insight
Arthritis, menstrual problems, digestive problems, skin conditions, asthma, muscular-skeletal problems, and pain relief....

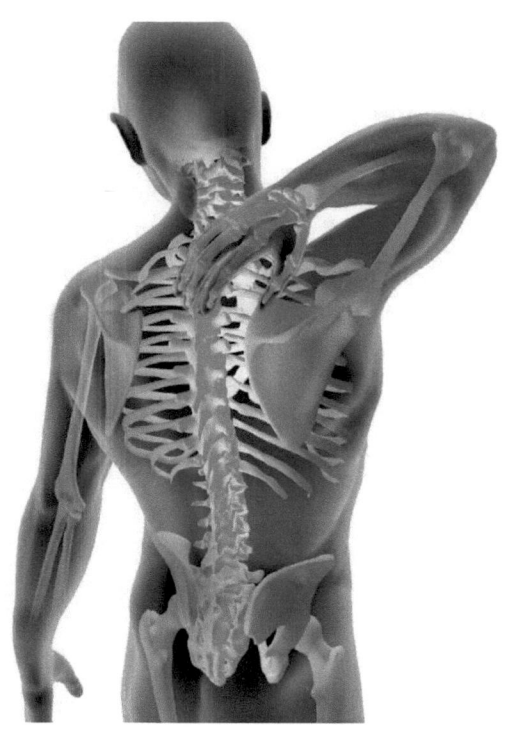

- Increased oxygenation of the blood
- Muscle toning throughout the body
- A clearer and more relaxed mind
- Improved posture
- Improved circulation of blood and lymph
- Regulation of bodily functions.

Heinz Duthel

Discover Complementary Healthcare

What is it? The easiest, simplest thing in the world -
with it comes great insight

Bibliografische Information der Deutschen Nationalbibliothek:
Die Deutsche Nationalbibliothek verzeichnet diese
Publikation in der Deutschen Nationalbibliografie;
detaillierte bibliografische Daten sind im Internet
über http://dnb.dnb.de abrufbar.

© 2017 Heinz Duthel

Illustration: Schriftsteller.club
Dritte Ausgabe 2017 – Third Edition 2017

Herstellung und Verlag: BoD – Books on Demand,
Norderstedt
ISBN: 9783744893428

9 783744 893428

Discover Complementary Healthcare

What is it? The easiest, simplest thing in the world - with it comes great insight

Arthritis, menstrual problems, digestive problems, skin conditions, asthma, muscular-skeletal problems, and pain relief....

Increased oxygenation of the blood

Muscle toning throughout the body

A clearer and more relaxed mind

Improved posture

Improved circulation of blood and lymph

Regulation of bodily functions.

Acupressure
Kahuna Bodywork
(Or Hawaiian Massage, Lomi Lomi)
Acupuncture

Kanpo
Alexander Technique

Kinesiology
Anthroposophical Medicine

Life-coaching
Aromatherapy

Manual Lymphatic Drainage (MLD)
Art Therapy

Massage Therapy
Aura Soma

McTimoney Chiropractic
Autogenic Training

Medau Movement
Ayurveda

Meditation
Bach Flower Remedies

Metabolic Typing
Bates Method

Metamorphic Technique
Biochemic Tissue Salts

Naturopathy
Biofeedback

Neuro Linguistic Programming (NLP)
Biorhythms

Norris Technique
Bowen Technique

Nutritional Therapy
Buteyko Technique

Osteopathy
Chiropractic

Pilates
Cognitive and Behavior Therapies

Polarity Therapy
Colonic Irrigation

Psychotherapy
Color Therapy

Qi Gong
Cranial Osteopathy

Radionics
Craniosacral Therapy

Reflexology
Do In

Reiki Healing
Ear Acupuncture

Rolfing
Emotional Freedom Technique

Seichem
Feldenkrais Method

Seiki
Feng Shui

Shiatsu
Flower Essences

Sound Therapy
Healing

Thai Foot Massage
Hellerwork

Thai Yoga Massage
Herbal medicine

The Journey
Holographic Repatterning

Thought Field Therapy
Homoeopathy

Toyohari
Hopi Ear Candles

Trager Work
Hypnotherapy

Tuina
Indian Head Massage (IHM)

Yoga
Iridology

Zero Balancing

Massage Therapy

What is it?

Massage is a systematic, therapeutic stroking and kneading of the soft tissues of the body. The word is derived from the Greek 'masso', to knead and the Arabic 'mass', to press gently. It has been used as a form of therapy for thousands of years and touch is the most instinctive response to pain. Touch is an essential requirement for healthy development in early life and research has shown the babies who have received massage from their mothers have increased weight gain, increased nerve and brain cell development and better hormonal functioning and cell activity. Earliest records of the use of massage as a therapy come from China over 5,000 years ago. The use of massage in the West became more popular in the 16th Century when a French doctor, Ambroise Pare incorporated a more anatomical and physiological approach. A Swede, Per Henrik Ling, developed a system of massage and gymnastics in the early 19th Century which became what we now know as Swedish massage. There are many different types of massage that have been developed; some approaches focus on the physical effects that the massage techniques have on the body, whilst others focus attention on the flow of 'energy' within the body. All types of massage can have an effect on the skin, muscles, blood vessels, lymph, nerves and some of the internal organs.

How Does Massage Work?

The relationship between the exterior and interior of the body is closely interlinked via the nervous system and it has been found that by stimulating specific areas on the surface of the body can have a corresponding effect on the internal organs and systems of the body. The dermis layer of the skin contains nerve endings which respond to touch and, on stimulation, the receptor nerves relay impulses via the spinal cord back to the brain. The brain then relays messages back to the area involved. The effects may include the relaxation of voluntary muscles, the sedation of nerve sensors and improved blood circulation to the area. The receptor nerve endings affected by touch travel more quickly than those involved in chronic pain and can reduce the brain's perception of the amount of pain from the affected area. Chemicals known as endorphins are also released from the brain and act as the body's natural painkillers. These help to counter the sensation of chronic pain and give a feeling of well-being and relaxation.

The following gives a brief description of some of the various types of massage available:

Anma

This is a traditional Japanese massage that works tsubos or acupressure points on the body. Anma became the basis of energy-based body techniques like shiatsu, tuina and Kahuna.

Aromatherapy

Aromatherapy is the combination of healing massage with the medicinal properties of essential oils from plant extracts. The essential oils are absorbed through the skin during massage and also by inhalation through the nose.

Aston Patterning

Developed in America by Judith Aston and has its roots in Rolfing, Aston Patterning is a system of massage, soft tissue bodywork, fitness training and movement education. It can be helpful in alleviating pain and improving posture by encouraging fluid body movements and even distribution of body weight.

Ayurvedic Massage

This is the massage aspect of Ayurvedic medicine. It is based on affecting the flow of 'prana' through the 107 'marma' points on the body. This is very similar to the approach used by Oriental Medicine as in Acupuncture. Depending on the constitution and the 'dosha type' of the client according to the principles of Ayurvedic Medicine, suitable oils are chosen to be used in the massage. There is also a form of massage for self-use.

Biodynamic Massage

Developed in the 1960's by a Norwegian physiotherapist and psychologist, Gerda Boyesen. The therapy aims to release energy believed to be trapped in the muscles and gut causing physical and emotional pain. Techniques can be soothing or more vigorous and Swedish massage is used together with other methods like 'lifting' the limbs to free trapped 'bio-energy' which is then released via the abdomen. Discussion is encouraged if the treatment raises any issues.

Chavutti Thirumal

Chavutti Thirumal comes from southern India and is part of the Ayurvedic system. It is said to have developed to promote suppleness to traditional dancers and martial art practitioners and is regarded as a specialized form of massage to aid the circulation, lymphatic system and digestion. The therapist is suspended above the client using a rope, and uses his or her feet and toes to apply firm, continuous strokes to stimulate the body's energy lines.

Hellerwork

Developed by Joseph Heller, an American engineer and Rolfing Practitioner, in the 1970's, it could be described as a blend of Rolfing, Alexander Technique and the Feldenkrais Method. It has three components: bodywork, movement education and verbal dialogue. The bodywork is a deep massage to the fascia which is where Joseph Heller believes stiffness and tension accumulate.

Indian Head Massage (Champissage)

Traditionally practiced in India to the head and hair in order to keep hair lustrous and healthy, it has been extended and enhanced to include deep and relaxing massage to the upper back, shoulders and neck which is an area susceptible to the build-up of tension. It helps to relax the thin layer of muscle covering the head, improving blood flow, nourishing the hair follicles and alleviating anxiety and stress.

Kahuna

An ancient Hawaiian system of massage that aims to help clients accept their own body and love themselves. Connection to one's own self-love is believed to strengthen the ability to recognize the beauty in our life and surroundings. The treatment involves the practitioner using long rhythmical strokes over a two hour period with the client lying naked on a treatment table. The massage increases the vibrational rate of the cells of the body.

Lomi

A deep tissue massage based on a Hawaiian Kahuna tradition.

Manual Lymphatic Drainage

A very light pressure massage is used on the skin to encourage and stimulate the superficial lymphatic system in order to assist the removal of toxins from the body via the lymphatic nodes. Dietary correction can also be advisable.

Remedial Massage

This is a corrective massage to encourage muscular alignment to muscle groups that are strained from overuse. The massage is deep and specific, concentrating on the muscles that are tight and stiff.

Rolfing

Rolfing (or Structural Integration) is a system of manipulation designed to bring the body into correct alignment.

Sports Massage

This is ideal for loosening muscle groups to regain flexibility and prevent strains occurring. It focuses on muscle recovery rate and helps to cleanse the muscles of toxins allowing less muscle fatigue after exercise. Deep massage is applied to the muscle groups.

Thai Massage

Thai massage is a blend of Chinese and Ayurvedic systems. It uses gentle stretching, bending and pulling techniques to affect the flow of 'prana' or vital force in the body. Treatment is focused on the massage channels and points on the body and a practitioner will use hands, feet and elbows to affect this flow and help to restore harmony to the body.

Therapeutic Massage (Swedish massage)

Is the manipulation of the soft tissues (skin, muscles, tendons and ligaments) of the body. It is a firm massage and has a set routine of techniques that vary from deep pressure to stimulate the body's systems, to a slower, more superficial movement to assist relaxation. There are four basic movements used in Therapeutic Massage:

Effleurage: relaxes and stretches the superficial muscles of the body.

Petrissage: kneading and squeezing of superficial and deeper muscles and soft tissue.

Friction: breaks down adhesions between tissues and relaxes muscle fibers.

Tapotement: a variety of percussive strokes to stimulate skin and muscles to increase blood flow.

Zero Balancing

It was developed in the 1970's by Dr Fritz Smith, an American doctor, osteopath and acupuncturist and is a touch technique that combines Eastern and Western medicine. Treatment aims to restore a smooth flow of energy throughout the body paying attention to 'foundation' joints that act as shock absorbers for the weight distribution of the body and to breathing patterns, eye movements and stomach rumbles. The improvement to the energy flow can help to improve posture, increase harmony and the bodies own self-healing ability. The practitioner uses gentle touch via the fingers to stretch and hold the client, who lies fully clothed on a treatment table.

Acupressure

What is it?

Acupressure is the application of pressure to the body to affect the flow of energy (Ki) in the 12 meridians according to the principles of Oriental medicine. It is widely practiced in China where more emphasis is given to a person's responsibility for their own health than it is in the West, and is often used as a self-help treatment.

Acupressure is believed to be the 'mother of Acupuncture' in that it predates the use of needles to stimulate the body's energy flow. It has the same principles as Acupuncture, but the pressure is applied directly to the Acupoints of the body mainly by using the hands, fingers, thumb or knuckles and sometimes by using a smooth, blunt object. Stimulation of the body's meridian system by touch is perhaps one of the oldest healing systems, and many other therapies use Acupressure techniques including Shen Tao, Jin Shen, Do Jin Shen, Qigong, Shiatsu and Tuina.

Acupuncture

What is it?

Acupuncture is an ancient Chinese medical procedure involving insertion and manipulation of needles at more than 360 points in the human body. Applied to relieve pain during surgery or in rheumatic conditions, and to treat many other illnesses, acupuncture is used today in most hospitals in China and by some private practitioners in Japan, Europe, and the United States.

Acupressure, a variant in which the practitioner uses manipulation rather than penetration to alleviate pain or other symptoms, is in widespread use in Japan and has begun to find adherents in the United States and elsewhere. Also known as shiatsu, acupressure is administered by pressing with the fingertips-and sometimes the elbows or knees-along a complex network of trigger points in the patient's body.

In traditional Chinese medicine, it is believed an energy called chi flows along invisible energy channels called 'meridians' which are believed to be linked to internal organs. Sticking needles at particular points along those meridians is believed to increase or decrease that flow of energy.

Chinese traditional medicine sees that a balance has to be kept between two opposing yet complementary natural forces called 'yin' (female) and 'yang' (male). Yin force is seen as being passive, tranquil, and represents darkness, coldness, moisture and swelling. Yang force is seen as being aggressive and stimulating, and represents light, heat, dryness and contraction.

History

Acupuncture needles dating from 4,000 years ago have been found in China. The first needles were made of stone; later, bronze, gold, or silver were used, and, today, needles are usually made of steel. Initially, needles were used only to prick boils and ulcers. Acupuncture was developed in response to the theory that there are special "meridian points" on the body connected to the internal organs, and that "vital energy" flows along the meridian lines. According to this theory, diseases are caused by interrupted energy flow and inserting and twirling needles restores normal flow.

Treatment

The primary use of acupuncture in China today is for surgical analgesia (pain relief). Chinese surgeons estimate that 30 per cent of surgical patients obtain adequate analgesia with acupuncture, which is now done by sending an electrical current through the needles rather than by twirling them. American doctors who have observed surgery done under acupuncture have verified that it is effective in some patients, but put the figure closer to 10 per cent. Brain surgery is especially amenable to this form of analgesia. Chinese surgeons claim that acupuncture is superior to Western, drug-induced analgesia in that it does not disturb normal body physiology, and, therefore, does not make the patient vulnerable to shock (acute fall in blood pressure).

Chinese doctors also treat some forms of heart disease with acupuncture. As part of an attempt to put the practice on a more scientific basis, they studied the effects of acupuncture treatment on more than 600 people with chest pain caused by reduced blood flow to the heart. They claimed that almost all the patients greatly reduced their use of medicine, and that most were able to resume work. Other physiological conditions treated with acupuncture are peptic ulcers, hypertension (high blood pressure), appendicitis, and asthma.

In 1979, the World Health Organization listed some 40 diseases that could be successfully treated with acupuncture, including breathing difficulties, digestive problems, disorders of the nervous system and painful menstruation

Alexander Technique

What is it?

The Alexander Technique is used to help to teach people about how efficiently and effortlessly they can use their bodies in everyday life. Often, we develop bad posture and habits without being aware of this, and expend too much energy or muscle force to achieve a task. Alexander Technique teachers help to adjust the client's posture to recognize the difference between current habits and what it feels like to use muscles with minimum effort and in a relaxed, fluid way. The Technique teaches how to become more aware of your own posture, balance and movement in everyday life.

The lessons usually last for between 30 and 45 minutes and are normally on a one-to-one basis. The teacher uses his/her hands to gently correct any muscular imbalances and encourages the body to a better alignment. This is a direct body experience, so the client becomes familiar with the sensation of correct alignment in their own body. This can feel strange initially, as the body is not used to using its muscles in this way, and the new methods of movement need to be practiced with constant awareness as to how we choose to use our bodies in everyday tasks. It is a process of re-educating the body by learning how to stand and move correctly. This leads to health benefits as often poor spinal posture will lead to other symptoms like poor breathing due to restriction in the throat and diaphragm areas. Breathing and how we breathe is an important aspect of the Alexander Technique.

The Alexander Technique was developed by an Australian actor, Frederick Matthias Alexander (1869-1955). He suffered from respiratory problems as a child, which later affected his voice and career in the theatre. He tried many remedies without success and eventually began a process of self-observation to try to find a way of curing himself. He realized that the voice problem was a result of muscular tension in his whole body and that his thought patterns also had a great part in contributing to the tension that had become an ingrained habit. Alexander studied his posture with the aid of mirrors to see how this was affected when he recited and as a result could see that his body alignment was incorrect. He gradually taught himself to correct his posture and found that he had cured his voice problem. He went on to pass the technique to others and eventually opened a clinic to help people to learn about their own use of posture.

Anthroposophical Medicine

An Austrian - Rudolf Steiner founded the philosophy of Anthroposophical Medicine in the early 1900's. Steiner's aim was to complement and develop medicine as it existed, rather than set up an alternative system. Together with Dr Ita Wegman, he developed his ideas to include a medical science, as well as his own principle of polarity.

The Seven Principles of Anthroposophical Medicine

Spirit manifests both within the human organism and outside of it in the substances of the kingdoms of nature.

The wisdom that created nature is also at work within the human being.

Anthroposophical Medicine is a leading holistic health movement throughout Europe and has been on the cutting edge of preserving therapeutic freedom in the public and legal realm.

Man has a divinely guided individual destiny, which includes individual freedom with the potential for error and illness.

Art is an indispensable part of human life. Out of AM, specialized disciplines of Therapeutic Eurythmy, Rhythmical Massage, clay modeling, painting and music therapy have evolved.

Remedies are derived from substances of the mineral, plant or animal kingdom. They can be prepared homeopathically, alchemically or as whole substance. They can be given orally, by injection or through external application.

Every treatment aims to enhance the life force of the patient as an axis for improved health and deepened self-knowledge.

What to expect

An anthroposophical doctor will ask questions about diet, lifestyle and constitution, with an emphasis on the body's rhythms - eating, sleeping and menstrual patterns. The doctor may also carry out standard medical tests, and will use the information to aid diagnosis, prescribing treatment to balance the poles and systems regulating the body.

Practitioners are fully qualified doctors, who make use of modern technology and medication as required - they consider that this approach gives them a fuller picture of an individual, allowing them to take a broader view of illness and therapy.

Because AM is a holistic system, aimed at harmonizing elements of the spiritual, as well as the physical self, it is said by its followers to be of benefit in cases where a conventional cure cannot be achieved.

Aromatherapy

What is Aromatherapy?

The art of applying essential oils to suit individual needs. The oils work directly on the chemistry of the body, via the skin and bloodstream.

Essential oils are extracts that contain the substances that give plants their smell. They are produced by tiny glands in the petals, leaves, stems, bark and wood of many plants and trees. In nature, they are released slowly, but when heated or crushed, their oil glands burst, releasing the plant's aroma more strongly.

It isn't known exactly when or where the art of aromatherapy began. It is thought that Chinese knowledge of medicinal oils may have reached the west by way of the Egyptians, Greeks and Roman. The first recorded use of plants in Britain was in the 13th century and from then on, manufacture increase and the oils became widely used as perfumes, antiseptics and medicines.

How are the oils applied?

Usually by massage, they can be given as a relaxing treatment covering "stress" areas such as back, shoulders, face, legs.

Essential oils can also be inhaled, using an oil burner or breathing in an infusion and can also be very beneficial when added to baths.

Who can it help?

Aromatherapy is believed to be suitable for people of all ages, even babies. Aroma therapists claim that they can treat many conditions, and often see a great improvement in nervous disorders, such as depression, anger, stress and other related symptoms such as headaches and insomnia.

Practitioners say that aromatherapy is safe for home use, but the following general guidelines should be observed:

Only high quality oils should be bought from a specialist aromatherapy supplier.

Pure oils should not be applied directly to the skin.

Oils should not be swallowed unless they are supplied by a fully trained aroma therapist and used under his/her supervision.

Some oils are to be avoided by pregnant women. Check with a trained aroma therapist.

Art Therapy

The use of art has always been used for self-expression and to convey ideas and emotions that are difficult to describe verbally. It's potential as a therapeutic tool became apparent after World War 2 when survivors of the war used art in hospitals and rehabilitation centers to help to overcome the traumas they had experienced.

What is Art Therapy?

Art Therapy is a non-verbal way of revealing deeper emotions that may not otherwise be clearly expressed. A form of psychotherapy where art (creative expression using various media: painting, drawing, sculpture etc.) is used to allow safe expression of emotions. The client is encouraged to express themselves freely through art, allowing a link between the subconscious the product of the art therapy. The resulting images can help to bring to light any suppressed emotions or conflicts. Reflecting on the images can help to understand and deal with the issues that arise. Art Therapy is also used as a tool for personal growth and greater self-understanding.

There are two main approaches to Art Therapy. One is that the act of creating the artwork is therapeutic in it and allows the client to understand their own inner conflicts and emotions without any interpretation from the therapist. The other approach takes the view that the artwork is a non-verbal method of communicating and allows the therapist to understand and identify the client's needs through interpretation to help them to deal with the issues.

Art Therapy is often used in hospitals, prisons, education centers and mental health clinics and is suitable for people of all ages. It is especially beneficial for emotional and psychological disorders as it provides a means of communication to express feelings that are too difficult to verbalize. It is also of great use for personal development and growth by helping to identify problem areas and then transform negative images into positive ones.

Therapy sessions may be on a one-to-one basis or in a group. An initial consultation is taken to determine general health, medical treatment and lifestyle details before any sessions commence. No previous art experience is necessary as the purpose is to use the art media to help to communicate deeper inner emotions which can then be self-interpreted.

Aura Soma

What is it

Aura-Soma is a form of color therapy. It was developed in 1984 by Vicky Wall, a UK chiropodist who developed psychic powers after losing her sight. She described Aura-Soma as "non-intrusive, self-selective soul therapy".

The remedies are a collection of small bottles, each containing a layer of colored essential oil on top of a layer of colored spring water containing herbal extracts. There are over 90 bottles in all and most of them contain two colors each. You are asked to choose the four colors that most appeal to you. The four that you choose are the most relevant to your physical and emotional condition and by applying the combination of colors to your skin daily, allows the body to absorb the colors and rebalance the body. There is no standard duration of treatment and the therapy is used as often as it is felt necessary.

Autogenic Training

What is it?

Autogenic Training is a form of self-hypnosis that aims to induce a state of relaxation and wellbeing, and to utilize the body's own healing power. Its originator was Dr Johannes Shultz, a psychiatrist and neurologist, who was strongly influenced by Professor Oscar Vogt, who had dedicated high life to psychosomatic medicine. Shultz developed Vogt's theory that patients who practiced simple verbal exercises to induce hypnosis could alleviate many physical and mental ailments.

Dr Shultz went on to develop a series of six Standard Autogenic Formulae - which still form the core of Autogenic Training and Therapy today. A book was published in 1932, and the training of teacher grew from there.

Autogenic Training is taught one to one, or in groups of 6 - 8, over a period of 8 weeks. The aim of the technique is to induce a balance between the two hemispheres of the brain, as well as between the two branches - sympathetic and parasympathetic - of the autonomic nervous system. It aims to give the student the power to induce physical and mental relaxation from within.

Extensive research has been carried out on the technique, and in some areas it is available on the

National Health Service. It is said to be effective for a myriad of conditions ranging from high blood pressure to ME, depression and addictions.

Ayurveda

What is it?

Ayurveda is most certainly the most ancient of all medical systems. It has its origins in India, and is still the most important form of medicine in the Indian subcontinent; its philosophies are also gaining ground in the West. Despite its antiquity, there are relatively few practitioners, particularly in the UK, due in part to the very length training and the huge complexity of its philosophy and teaching. Classical Ayurvedic training is conducted in Sanskrit. Most Ayurvedic practitioners tend to be orthodox doctors as well.

The word 'Ayurveda' comes from Sanskrit and means 'the science of life', the whole aim of Ayurveda is prevention. The ancient texts say that the human lifespan should be around 100 years, and that all those years should be lived in total health, both physical and mental, therefore the Ayurvedic practitioner is looking to balance the body and mind, find health problems before they occur or arrest them before they do any real harm. It is a complete philosophical and spiritual system, which has over thousands of years become subtle, sophisticated and highly complex. However, the basic tenets are reasonably easy to understand and have changed little over the centuries.

The five elements - ether, air, fire, water and earth are the foundations on which the Ayurvedic interpretation of all matter and life is based, they are not to be interpreted literally however, each represents qualities and different types of force and energy, as well as some form of physical manifestation. The elements do not act in isolation - three different combinations of the elements, called tridosha, are what form the basis for diagnosis, treatment, cure and health maintenance in Ayurvedic medicine. Each individual's constitution is determined by the state of their parents' doshas at the time of conception, and upon birth a person has the levels of the three doshas that is right for them. Life and all its forces can cause the doshas to become unbalanced which can lead to ill health.

Each of the three doshas has a role to play in the body:

VATHA is the driving force, it relates mainly to the nervous system and the body's energy center.

PITTA is fire, it relates to the metabolism, digestion, enzymes, acid and bile.

KAPHA is related to Water in the mucous membranes, phlegm, moisture, fat and lymphatics.

What to expect

There is no typical Ayurvedic session - even the methods of diagnosis may vary from practitioner to practitioner. The basic diagnosis is known as the three-point diagnosis and involves detailed observation of your appearance, examination by touch, and a detailed questionnaire about your life and health. After diagnosis comes treatment, and the range of treatments is vast, however, you will be given guidelines for healthy living and instructed in the diet, which will soothe and correct imbalances in your body type. You may be prescribed a course of purification to eliminate toxins from the body and to energize the body's elimination mechanisms. Herbal preparations may be prescribed. A host of other healing techniques including massage, exercise, breathing and meditation may be used.

Bach Flower Remedies

What is it?

The term 'Flower Remedy' refers to the products developed by Dr Edward Bach, a London bacteriologist and homoeopath. 'Flower Essences' are products devised by various people following on from Dr Bach's work.

Dr Bach became disillusioned with the side effects of drug therapies and turned his research to the healing power of nature. He believed that illness was a result of mental or emotional balance and that the unique energetic property of a plant could be used to rectify an imbalance and restore the awareness of 'wholeness'. Using the homoeopathic law of potentization, he reasoned that the healing effects of plants might also be contained in the morning dew found on their flowers.

Dr Bach believed that harmful emotions were the main cause of disease and he classified the various emotions into seven main categories. These seven categories were then divided further into 38 negative feelings. Each negative emotion is associated with a particular plant. He also developed a compound of five flowers called Rescue Remedy to be used in emergency situations or for trauma.

The Seven Emotional Categories and Sub-Categories

Fearfulness

    Terror and nightmares
    Known fears and shyness
    Uncontrollable rage and impulses
    Vague fears and apprehension
    Excessive fear on behalf of family and friends

Uncertainty

    Lack of confidence in decision making
    Indecision and mood swings
    Hesitation and past disappointments
    Despair and hopelessness
    Tiredness and procrastination

Dissatisfaction and lack of motivation

Lack of interest in present circumstances

Lack of concentration and escapism
Nostalgia and homesickness
Apathy and resignation
Lack of vitality and exhaustion
Worry
Melancholy
Failure to learn from mistakes

Loneliness

Aloofness and reserve
Impatience
Self-obsession, self-absorption and excessive desire for companionship

Over-sensitivity

Concealed problems
Anxiety to please
Periods of transition
Negative feelings such as hatred or envy

Despondence and despair

Lack of self-confidence
Guilt and self-reproach
Sense of overwhelming responsibility
Unbearable anguish

Shock and grief
Resentment and bitterness
Losing the strength to fight
Feeling ashamed or unclean

Over-concern for welfare of others

Possessiveness, selfishness, self-pity and over-protectiveness towards others
Argumentative and overbearing
Ruthless and dictatorial
Critical and intolerant
Self-denial and narrow-mindedness

Flower Remedies and Essences are liquid preparations created by boiling parts of plants in spring water or by placing the flowers onto the surface of spring water and leaving them to infuse by natural sunlight for a period of time. After these processes, the water is preserved in brandy. Bach Flower Remedies are made of flowers found mostly in Britain.

The Remedies are intended for self-help use, although many practitioners from other disciplines also prescribe their use. The Remedies are sold in concentrated form and the method of use is either by placing drops directly on the tongue, or by diluting them in liquid.

Bates Method

What is it?

The Bates method is a holistic approach to vision which concentrates on the use of the mind rather than the eyes. Surgery and lenses are considered counterproductive as they treat the symptoms rather than the cause of defective vision, which is strain. The principle of re-education is similar to that used in Alexander Technique. There is also an emotional aspect, and practitioners may recommend Bach flower remedies, homoeopathy, or similar ways to address this.

Dr William H. Bates (1860-1931) was an American ophthalmologist who found that the relief of mental strain was fundamental to good use of the eyes. We need to reverse habits of strain (which are mainly unconscious) and take on board a new attitude to the world around us.

A practitioner will assess what you see and how you see it, and then work with you using the basic techniques in ways that are relevant to yourself. As you experience changes, you will be able to incorporate the techniques into your daily life. Usually it will take six to twelve sessions to teach you these, but may take longer in some cases.

The main techniques are:

Palming: cupping the hands over closed eyes to shut out any light and induce relaxation. Blinking is also good.

Shifting: practicing the awareness that any point you look at becomes most distinct when you look at it and less distinct when you look at a different point.

Swinging: developing awareness of movement in all areas of the visual field, even when you are the only thing moving.

Working with memory and imagination.

Biochemic Tissue Salts

What is it?

In the 19C Dr Wilhelm Heinrich Schussler identified twelve minerals that he believed to be vital to human health. Schussler was a German doctor of medicine, who was also a biochemist and homeopath.

Biochemic Tissue Salts are these twelve minerals in homeopathically prepared formulations, which are highly diluted. The salts are taken in the form of small tablets, dissolved under the tongue. Common symptoms treated with the salts include colds, catarrh, coughs, hay fever, headaches, indigestion and minor skin conditions.

Homeopaths, naturopaths and herbalists will often recommend tissue salts as part of a nutritional programme, but they are also frequently used as a self-help measure. Many health shops and some chemists, especially homeopathic pharmacies, stock the salts, and manufacturers usually provide dosage information.

Biofeedback

Biofeedback helps people regulate some aspect of their body by using signals from the body. The essence of Biofeedback training, as of all learning and training, is Knowledge of Results; Biofeedback instruments tell you what is happening in one or another part of your body, so you can regulate it better and feel better.

There is a variety of kinds of instruments, from simple to complex, of prices, from below £100 to many thousands ££, and of help or training needed to start using the instruments, from Nil to some days.

Biofeedback has been used for more than a generation by clinics, hospitals, many kinds of therapist and by individuals who feel better for using it, or who are exploring their personal growth and development.

What is Biofeedback?

Biofeedback instruments come in several kinds. They all connect to the body and provide a signal back to the user, often a sound or a meter reading or a computer graphic, which tells the user what is going on in that part of their body.

Biofeedback does not change you, you change, using the information from the instrument. If you don't want to change, don't waste your time with Biofeedback.

How does Biofeedback work?

It's simple; Biofeedback instruments tell you what is going on, and you can use what they tell you to improve your control of that aspect of your body's working.

To take a popular example, people can learn to improve the way they respond to stress by using instruments like the Relaxometer and the GSR2 to regulate their 'Fight or Flight' reaction when they come under stress. This reflex reaction produces a group of changes that we don't usually notice, including a rise in the electrical conductance of the skin. (If the stress is really severe you may break out in a sweat, all over! This is an extreme example of that kind of change.)

These instruments measure the change and produce a sound (and maybe a meter reading) which tells you at once when you get more upset or tense and when you relax, even a little bit.

By practising in a quiet place, and rehearsing in your mind stressful situations that you have faced (or might face) you can learn how to relax quickly, and so how to manage yourself better in the stressful situations. Then you can apply what you have learned even when you are not using the instrument.

You have learned the skill of calming down and use it when you need it.

Anyone can do this, including children and very old people, without the need for a therapist. Where someone has developed a complex and long-standing problem they may need the help of a psychologist or other professional therapist.

Are there other kinds of Biofeedback?

Yes, there are many; in fact is seems likely that if a person can get immediate knowledge of changes in some part of their body they can learn to regulate that part of the body. But only some of the successful research results have been taken up by therapists.

Many Physiotherapy and Occupational Therapy departments of hospitals use feedback of muscle tension. While you may be well able to tense or relax a muscle when you want to, people who have had a stroke, or been born with cerebral palsy, or been injured in an accident, can't make their muscles do what they want. Some (but not all) of these people can learn to improve control of their muscles again. And they improve more with Biofeedback than without - there is a large body of research literature about it.

This type of feedback is called Electro-Myo-Graphic feedback, or EMG. Very effective work on managing urinary incontinence in women has been done with EMG Biofeedback.

Some people learn a pattern of responding in their muscles to stressful situations. If this is sustained it can become painful, and then it is useful to apply EMG feedback to learning to relax the tense muscles. 'Stiff Neck' pain and writer's cramp can be relieved in this way.

Migraine headaches respond very well to Biofeedback training in relaxation, either by training in finger-warming, or just using the skin conductance feedback described above.

Feedback of brain electrical activity, EEG, has been available for many years. The brain rhythm called Alpha occurs more in people meditating than when they are not meditating, and many people use EEG feedback to enhance their meditative state. Alpha activitiy also seems to be incompatible with anxiety, and so training in Alpha activity has been used in hospitals to help deal with chronic anxiety.

There is a growing interest in training EEG patterns in children to help them with Attention Deficit Disorder and in working with adults with substance abuse problems in a similar way. This involves expensive computer systems and does require a trained therapist. It offers the prospect of training a person to produce some partcular sort of EEG patterns which are associated with a particular psychological state, and will be a very exciting area for further work.

Don't let anyone tell you 'Scientists don't understand how Biofeedback works...' It is like learning to talk. You know you are speaking right when you talk like the people around you; you are using auditory feedback to do this, and deaf people can't have that feedback so they need help learning to talk. With feedback you get better at speaking.

With feedback from your bathroom scales you can learn you are losing weight; with feedback from his mirror and his partner :-) a man learns to shave properly. This feedback or knowledge of results is essential to all learning. Biofeedback applies the principle to learning to control your body, and leads to control of aspects that used to be thought of as 'just automatic' but actually can be altered, like blood pressure and heart rate. But it only works if you, the user, want to change.

There is a great deal of successful work on managing high blood pressure (BP). It is particularly relevant to use Biofeedback if there seems to be a psychological component to the high BP, and much less so if there is a clear medical condition, such as kidney failure, causing the high BP.

What else may Biofeedback help with?

The list of ailments which have been helped by Biofeedback is long. About 20 appear below. There is a longer list (with some duplication) on the web site of the professional body: Association for Applied Psychophysiology and Biofeedback, www.aapb.org

and then look at Potential Clients. This site is an important source of information about the field.

Anxiety, Back ache, Blushing, Bruxism, Clammy hands, Dysmenorrhea, Headache, High Blood Pressure, Migraines, Muscle spasms, Paralysis, Phobia, Raynaud's syndrome, Spasticity, Sleep problems, Stammering, Stiff neck, Stress, Tension headaches, TMJ Syndrome, Trouble with people (boss, family etc.)

If you study Meditation learning to control brain electrical activity (EEG) will be of interest to you.

There are many more kinds of Biofeedback, and uses for them, though some of them are awkward to use or are only anecdotal and have not become accepted practice.

Some idea of the extent of sound scientific research about Biofeedabck can be obtained from the site of the Association for Applied Psycho- physiology and Biofeedback mentioned above: www.aapb.org

There is a substantial peer-reviewed quarterly scientific Journal about work in the field, published continuously since 1975, titled "Applied Pshychophysiology And Biofeedback" and published by Kluwer Academic/Plenum Publishers in Dordrecht, Netherlands, and New York, USA. Many professional journals have published work on the application of Biofeedback to their particular field

Biorhythms

Many human functions follow a natural pattern of behaviour, from waking and sleeping in a 24 hour period, to the female menstrual cycle of 28 days. Biorhythm theory uses scientific methods to chart rhythms that affect the internal functioning of the body, particularly the physical, emotional and intellectual abilities.

What is it?

Biorhythm theory originated with research by two doctors in the early 20th century, both working independently of each other. Dr Hermann Swoboda, a psychologist at the University of Vienna, monitored his patient's emotional moods, dreams and physical symptoms over long periods. He noted in particular that asthma attacks recurred in a regular cycle and concluded that there were two distinct cycles of 23 and 28 days, which he termed 'physical' and 'emotional' respectively. Wilhelm Fleiss, an ear, nose and throat specialist in Berlin was also interested in biological cycles through analysis of his patient's medical records. His knowledge of numerology together with his record analysis led him to the conclusion that the numbers 23 and 28 had significance to many bodily functions. He described the two cycles as 'solar' (masculine) at 23 days and 'lunar' (feminine) at 28 days.

The combined work of Swoboda and Fleiss was developed further in the 1920's by an Austrian mathematician and engineer, Alfred Teltscher. He studied the intellectual rhythms of his students and found a 33 day cycle which he called the 'intellectual' cycle.

Further work has revealed other cycles, namely a 38 day intuitive cycle, a 43 day aesthetic cycle and a 53 day spiritual cycle.

In Biorhythm theory, the 3 main cycles of 23, 28 and 33 days are charted from birth, starting at zero. When illustrated as a graph, the three cycles rise from zero to a high point, descend back to the zero line and then fall correspondingly to a low point and back again to zero. As each cycle is a different length, they intersect each other occasionally. On the days when one or more of the cycles crosses the zero line, it is considered to be a 'critical' day when that particular cyclical functioning is low and the person can be prone to accidents or negative events.

Biorhythm charts are easily charted using computer software technology. It is used to assess when the optimum physical, emotional or intellectual peak is for a person and to be aware of the 'critical' times when some tasks may prove to be more difficult.

Bowen Technique

What is it?

The Bowen Technique is a gentle and non-invasive holistic treatment that aims to restore balance to the body by using small, gentle moves to specific areas of the body. Because the therapy is so gentle, it is considered to be suitable for all ages. The precise, light movements are applied either directly on the skin or through light clothing to the muscles, tendons or ligaments. A delicate, cross-fibre movement is used to release tension and energetic blocks held in the muscles, allowing the body to rebalance itself naturally and therefore maximise the potential for healing.

The technique was developed in Australia by Thomas A Bowen (1916-1982). Although he did not explain or document his theory of how the Bowen Technique worked, he did allow six apprentices to study his methods with him during his lifetime. Bowen continually developed his methods of treatment and as the apprentices studied with him at different times of the evolution of his therapy, this resulted in slightly different emphasis on the various methods by the students. Oswald Rentsch studied with Bowen for two and a half years and was commissioned by Bowen to teach the method to others. The Bowen Technique is now being taught and practised in Australia, North America, New Zealand, Europe and the United Kingdom.

The Treatment

A Bowen treatment usually takes place with the client lying on a couch or sitting in a chair. A practitioner uses his fingers and thumbs to 'roll' the muscles and connective tissue using gentle pressure at specific points. Many of the points used correspond to the trigger points used in massage or the acupressure points. The movements assist blood circulation and lymphatic drainage, helping to clear toxins from the body. A session usually lasts from half an hour to an hour with frequent pauses between movements to allow the body time to assimilate changes. The client is left to rest at the end of the treatment for the same reason.

Symptoms that may respond well to the Bowen Technique include back pain, sciatica, neck and shoulder problems, sports injuries, migraines and headaches, menstrual problems, chronic fatigue and stress related problems.

Buteyko Technique

The Buteyko breathing technique involves teaching people with breathing problems simple exercises using voluntary breath control, with the intention of reducing the frequency and severity of their symptoms.

The impetus behind this approach has come principally from the work of a Russian physician Dr Konstantin Buteyko, after whom the technique has been named. Although mainly centred on specific breathing exercises, the programme also pays attention to diet, physical exercise and emotional factors.

In May 2008 the updated British Guidelines for the Management of Asthma endorsed the Buteyko technique for the control of asthma symptoms, so that GPs and asthma nurses can now recommend it. The new guidelines grade the research on Buteyko as a 'B' classification - indicating that there are high quality clinical trials supporting the efficacy of the therapy in reducing both asthma symptoms and bronchodilator usage.

What is the Buteyko technique?

Buteyko is a system of breathing techniques based on clinical evidence that people with breathing problems tend to 'over-breathe'. The technique aims to restore the natural balance of breathing by teaching people how to breathe less. This is achieved by:

Learning to improve control over the respiratory muscles

Gradually increasing tolerance to the feeling of breathlessness

Understanding how external factors can affect breathing

Learning how to relax the muscles involved in breathing

The Buteyko technique is holistic in the sense that it tries to take into account all aspects of an individual's physical and mental condition within the context of their lifestyle, environment and diet.

What is the Buteyko technique commonly used for?

The Buteyko technique is used to improve the health of people with asthma and those with other breathing related problems such as COPD (chronic obstructive pulmonary disease), sinusitis, rhinitis, panic attacks and snoring.

Buteyko is used alongside other approaches, in particular conventional medicine.

The fundamental aim of Buteyko is to improve the quality of life of those suffering from breathing problems. In order to achieve the best possible results an individualised programme is taught, guided by the person's own aims.

What will happen when I see a Buteyko teacher?

A Buteyko teacher will guide you through the process of learning the breathing exercises and advise you on how best to manage your condition. Most people will need 4 - 6 sessions, each lasting around an hour, to fully understand and properly practise the techniques. The optimum frequency of lessons is weekly, but sessions may initially be more frequent.

On your first visit, your breathing and general health will be assessed. You will then be taught Buteyko techniques, graded according to your condition, aiming to help you to breathe in a relaxed effortless way. The lessons focus on learning and practicing these techniques.

The breathing techniques themselves are not physically demanding and the majority of the programme is carried out sitting comfortably in a chair. You will also be encouraged to undertake some form of regular daily exercise (such as walking) and to use particular breathing styles while you exercise.

If your teacher feels it is helpful, he or she may advise on changes to your diet to assist in restoring normal respiratory function.

For many people stress and emotion can play a part in bringing on symptoms. As part of the programme you will be taught techniques to quickly manage your breathing pattern. This can prevent the situation where anxiety and disordered breathing combine to make symptoms worse.

You will be asked to practise exercises at home between sessions; it is important to understand that if you do not do this practice you are much less likely to see improvements in your health. The good news is that by following the Buteyko programme the majority of people notice a significant improvement in their condition within a couple of weeks.

As Buteyko is about changing your breathing in everyday situations, no special clothing is necessary. Sometimes women prefer to wear trousers rather than a skirt.

What precautions should I take?

Please ensure your teacher is registered with the Buteyko Breathing Association (see below 'How do I find a Buteyko Teacher').

Your teacher will ask you to complete a confidential questionnaire, make sure you give details of past and present treatments for any medical problems. Buteyko is inherently safe, but there are some conditions where we would not advise using Buteyko at all; and other conditions where a cautious approach is required.

What will it cost?

The Buteyko technique is taught in some hospitals and GP surgeries.

Contact the Buteyko Breathing Association (BBA)

Chiropractic

What is it?

Chiropractic - from the Greek Chiropraktikos meaning "effective treatment by hand".

Chiropractic medicine was originally practiced in the late 19th Century by Daniel Palmer, a schoolteacher turned healer. Palmer's interest in healing lay in the cause of illness and he devoted much time to studying other cultures and races to see how they approached the problem. He was fascinated to learn that the ancient Egyptians had used spinal manipulation on displaced vertebrae to give relief from a wide variety of ailments. Palmer became increasingly interested in this, and began to develop his own methods of manipulation. After a number of successful treatments, he set up the first training institute to promote and further develop chiropractic medicine

What to expect...

Chiropractors' aim is to maintain the spine and nervous system in good health through neuromuscu-loskeletal manipulation. The same methods of consultation - case history, physical examination, labatory analysis and often x-rays are uniform through-out the industry.

A client will be asked to strip down to their underwear and posture will be studied whilst standing, sitting and lying down. Reflexes will be tested, and muscles palpated for signs of tension and spasm. Legs may also be measured to ascertain that they are of equal length. It is only after a thorough examination, that a chiropractor will decide if a problem is suitable for treatment. The aim of such treatment is to restore a full range of movement to the joints of the spine, relax and lengthen muscles, tendons and ligaments and relieve pain. Manipulation may be carried out by stretching muscles and short, controlled thrusts against a joint, also included in a treatment may be soft tissue techniques such as massage, heat, ice and kneading.

A treatment may last between 10-30 minutes, and generally a course will be prescribed to ensure maximum benefits are obtained. Chiropractors recommend the method for a variety of conditions ranging from chronic back trouble to migraine, ADD in children and many gynecological conditions. It does also have contraindications for a number of complaints such as osteoporosis, cancer and serious circulatory problems, so it is important to ensure that the practitioner is fully qualified and registered with a suitable governing body.

Cognitive and Behaviour Therapies

What is it?

Cognitive and Behaviour Therapies are the most studied and widely evaluated of the different psycho-therapeutic approaches. As well as being recognised by the medical profession as useful for treating many emotional and lifestyle problems, they are also wide-ly available in private, voluntary and government funded counselling agencies. They are the basis be-hind such services as marriage guidance, bereave-ment, post-traumatic stress and substance abuse counselling

Cognitive Therapy

An experienced psychotherapist will probably draw on several different types of CT - the underlying precept behind them all is that it is our perception of ourselves and others, and of the events that gave rise to them that cause emotional and behavioural prob-lems, and not the events themselves. The aim of the therapy is to alter a clients belief system in order that problems can be eliminated.

Brief Solution-Focused Therapy - this is generally the therapy used when a specific problem i.e. phobia, is present. It generally takes up to 3 sessions.

Cognitive-Analytical Therapy - This approach draws on psychoanalytic as well as cognitive tech-niques. A structured and focused framework is used to encourage patients to understand the origins of their attitudes and beliefs, and the effect they have on present feelings and behaviour in order that change may occur. Treatment may take several months or even longer.

Cognitive-Behavioural Therapy - psychologists rather than psychotherapists developed this method of treatment. Clients are required to question and remodel their basic outlook on life. Treatment may last from about three months.

Rational-Emotive Behaviour Therapy - Similar to CBT, practitioners of REBT believe that most emotional distress is the result of irrational or harmful beliefs. A technique called "disputing" is used to help patients to question their current attitudes and expectations, and to replace negative ones with new, more positive and productive ones.

Reality Therapy - Reality Therapists believe that human behaviour is designed to satisfy five basic needs, survival, the need to belong, the desire for power, the urge for freedom and the need for pleasure and entertainment. RT is designed to make people aware of their responsibility for their own actions and to recognise the failings of their current behaviour patterns and beliefs to satisfy their five basic needs, the client is then guided into exploring other ways of behaving and feeling. Treatment generally lasts for several months.

Personal Construct Therapy - PCT is based on the theory that we perceive the world not as it is, but as we construct it from personal experience. Treatment involves helping clients to restructure their view of the world, and is likely to last several months.

Behavioural Therapy

Behaviourism was an attempt to explain human psychology through studies of the behaviour of animals - Ivan Pavlov being the instigator. In the years after Pavlov's theory became common knowledge, a number of researchers began to apple the findings to the study of human behaviour.

Behavioural therapists believe that poorly adapted behaviour and negative attitudes feed back into the environment, making it worse and reinforcing the stimuli that caused the problems in the first place. The aim of the therapy is therefore to correct the undesirable behaviour patterns and perceptions, and to encourage the formation of behaviours and attitudes that are well adapted and productive.

Colour Therapy

What is colour therapy?

Colour therapy is based on the ancient art of using colour and light to treat disease.

Practitioners believe that by altering the colours that surround us, it is possible to enhance health and well-being

The earliest forms of therapy included the use of coloured gems and sunlight. There is now a wide range of treatment options available and many practitioners combine the use of colour with other complementary therapies such as aromatherapy, massage, reflexology, crystals and yoga.

What are the principles of colour therapy?

The human body absorbs light that is made up of the colour spectrum. Each colour in the spectrum has a frequency, wavelength and energy associated with it. The colours we absorb can have an effect on the nervous system, the endocrine system and subsequently on the release of hormones and other organic substances within the human body. They can also have an effect on the more subtle energies of the chakra system. This may affect our mental, emotional, psychological and physical states of health.

The symptoms of disease are a sign that there is a shortage of, or improper utilization of colour and light in the cells and organs of the human body. This may be due to factors such as our lifestyle, our environment, stress or too much, or too little of a particular colour frequency in our energy system. This imbalance can be corrected by the selective use of colour frequencies. The forms by which the frequencies of colour can be transmitted to the body are numerous.

What happens in a consultation?

An initial appointment will last about two hours. The practitioner will spend time finding out as much as possible about you, your medical history, and current physical health and state of mind.

The practitioner will identify the particular colour frequencies that you need. There are several ways of doing this including kinesiology to test muscle strength in relation to colour, dowsing and diagnostic charts in addition to the practitioner's own experience.

A typical colour therapy treatment might include the use of breathing exercises, crystals, light, silk scarves or coloured (solarised) water. Coloured light might be applied to parts or to the whole body. The main colour is usually given with its complementary colour (for example blue with orange). The lights may be used constantly or rhythmically.

You may be given advice on how to make the best use of colour in your diet, the clothes you wear and your home and work environment.

Which problems can colour therapy help?

Colour is used in orthodox medicine for the treatment of neonatal jaundice and other specific medical conditions. It is used in complementary therapy to boost the immune system and promote healing from within.

It can benefit a wide range of problems including stress-related conditions such as insomnia, anxiety, asthma, behavioural disorders and depression and many more. In particular, it can help to restore health after surgery or illness. It can also aid creativity and help learning.

How do I find a qualified colour therapist?

The majorities of colour therapists are self-employed and work, either from their own home or from a room rented in a natural health centre or clinic. When choosing a colour therapists, it is important to make sure that the practitioner has been properly trained at an accredited school or training establishment and is a member of a professional organisation. Practitioner members of the International Association of Colour use the letters PMIAC and are included in the Register of qualified practitioners which is sent out free of charge (on request only) to members of the public.

Cranial Osteopathy

What is it?

Cranial Osteopathy began in the early part of the 20th Century, its instigator was a man called William Garner Sutherland, who originally trained as an osteopath. Sutherland developed an interest in the cranium after recognizing that there was a rhythm in the cerebrospinal fluid surrounding the skull. Cerebrospinal fluid acts as protection for the brain, as well as supplying nutrients to, and draining waste products from it. In health, Sutherland found that there would be a regular pulse of between 12 and 15 beats per minute, and a disturbance of this pulse would indicate an imbalance somewhere in the body.

A Cranial Osteopath uses tiny, gentle manipulations to the skull, spinal column and sacral area, with the aim of restoring balance. Other areas of the body may also be added to achieve maximum results.

Conditions that Cranial Osteopathy claims to help include chronic migraine, asthma and allergies. It is also used more and more in the treatment of babies who have had difficult births.

Craniosacral Therapy

What is it?

Cranio-Sacral Therapy is a gentle form of holistic therapy developed from cranial osteopathy and oriental approach to bodywork. It uses touch to evaluate and affect the cranio-sacral system, i.e. the cranium (skull), the spinal column and the membranes and cerebrospinal fluid that surround and protect the brain and spinal cord. It is believed that changes in the cerebrospinal fluid will in turn affect every cell in the body via the connective tissue.

Dr John E Upledger, an American osteopath, developed cranio-sacral therapy from the cranial osteopathy work of Dr William Garner Sutherland. The key differences in Upledger's development of the therapy was to focus the treatment on the soft tissues, fluid and membrane of the cranio-sacral system rather than the bones, and that the rhythm of the cranio-sacral fluid was independent to the heart and respiration rates.

Treatment usually takes place on a couch with the client wearing light clothing. The practitioner will gently palpate areas of the body (usually the sacrum at the base of the spine and the head), using a very light touch to feel the cranial rhythmic impulse (CRI) of the cerebrospinal fluid. The treatment aim is to restore balance by allowing the removal of restrictions to the movement of the CRI to facilitate the body's own self-healing. A Cranio-Sacral session will normally last between 30 and 60 minutes and is suitable for everyone, including babies, children and the elderly.

Cranio-Sacral Therapy may help many conditions as it can affect all aspects of the body by enhancing general health, reducing stress and improving brain and spinal cord function. It is commonly used to treat conditions such as chronic pain, scoliosis, coordination problems, post-operative care, sports injuries, depression, birth trauma, hyperactivity and hormonal imbalances.

Do In
What is Do In?

Do In (also called Daoyin, Dao-In and Tao-In) is a self-help therapy that combines some of the principles of Shiatsu and Acupressure with stretches, exercises, breathing, meditation techniques and in some cases following a macrobiotic diet.

Do-In means self-stimulation in Japanese and refers to the various methods used to gather and strengthen energy (Ki) in the meridian systems of the body, especially in the abdominal area known as the Hara. Do-In also helps to eliminate toxins, promote self-development and increase spirituality. Contemplation and meditation are important aspects of a Do-In session to increase spiritual harmony and understanding.

Exercises used in a Do-In session:

Hara Breathing: methods of using the breath to centre the Ki in the Hara, or abdomen.

Self-Shiatsu Massage: a series of massage techniques to restore the flow of Ki along the meridians, using tapping, squeezing, rubbing and pressure to the whole body.

Makko-Ho Stretches: six stretches, very similar to Hatha Yoga postures, but designed to stimulate and rebalance the Ki along associated pairs of the 12 main Ki meridians in the body.

Meditation: methods of meditation and contemplation to quieten the mind and increase awareness and understanding.

Ear Acupuncture

What is it?

Ear Acupuncture is a wonderfully flexible therapy, that combines well with other treatments, and in which practitioners can be trained to a variety of different levels. Some colleges train their students in Ear Acupuncture alone, or in conjunction with Naturopathic or Chinese Medicine studies. However, practitioners can also be trained to administer the 5-needle drug detoxification protocol only (and this has been very effective for the training of staff that work in drug treatment centres).

Treatment is normally given with the patient sitting; hence the therapy lends itself equally well to treatment on a one to one basis; or to drop in clinics where patients may be treated as a group. This enables the therapy to be offered both privately or in charitably run clinics allowing it to be made available to the less well off.

Although Acupuncture has been around for as much as 5,000 years, Ear Acupuncture did not really take off until the 1950's when a French Physician Dr Paul Nogier noticed that some of his patients had healed scars from cauterisation for Sciatica. Some historians have suggested that the cauterisation technique was brought back from China by 16th century missionaries, but anyway he investigated further and his researches led him to develop a complete map of the ear. A report on his research was published in a European Acupuncture Journal in 1956, and came to the attention of Chinese researchers, who enthusiastically pursued this new speciality. Nogier's work was pioneering and his reflex maps are still in use today. He passed away in 1990, but is recognised as the 'Father' of modern ear Acupuncture.

At the time The Yellow Emperor's Classic was written in 500 BC only 6 ear points were known, those that connected the 6 Yang meridians to the auricle. Since then due to Nogier's pioneering work and continued research in China, Europe and the USA more than 200 usable points have been mapped and treatment protocols have been developed for a wide range of conditions. In addition to needling, treatment methods have been developed using ear seeds, magnets, electro stimulation and laser therapy.

The range of conditions for which treatment protocols have been developed includes: addictive behaviours including smoking, acute and chronic pain, some neurological conditions (including post Polio syndrome), stress related and psychological disorders, skin circulatory respiratory and digestive disorders.

Emotional Freedom Technique

What is EFT?

Emotional Freedom Technique (EFT) is an energy therapy that works on rebalancing the flow of energy that gets disrupted as it flows through the channels in your body known as "meridians". It was once thought that bad memories caused negative emotions but we now know that it's the disruption in your body's energy system that actually causes negative emotions, feelings and responses. What causes this energy disruption in some people and not in others can depend upon whether you were affected by a psychological or emotional trauma for instance or it could be the way you were brought up or conditioned to respond to negative events.

Imagine as a child you were locked in a dark cupboard as a punishment. As you grow up these associated fears and feelings could be "triggered" again at any time. This could be when you board a plane or when you go to the cinema. You may not even be consciously aware of how your fear of flying or being in a dark cinema has anything to do with being locked in a cupboard as a child.

Scientists recognise this "mind-body" connection but until now didn't know how to deal with it. On the other hand, the medical profession have been spending millions treating the symptoms of addiction, depression, anxiety, phobias etc with drugs that don't get to or treat the underlying cause. EFT helps to get to the root cause of the symptoms and deal with them.

How does it work?

EFT works by tapping on certain parts of your body whilst focusing on the problem and saying certain phrases. The idea is whilst focusing on the negative problem whilst tapping on those meridians nearest the surface of the skin, that the energy is rebalanced. For example, you would still remember being trapped in the cupboard, but after using EFT the associated fears and negative feelings would go and never (if rarely) return. The tapping routine takes about 1-2minutes to apply and can be used to overcome problems such as smoking, cravings, fear of flying, anxiety about exams, painful memories, low self esteem and even physical pain plus much more.

What happens during a session?

Usually the Practitioner will offer you a consultation to give you the opportunity to discuss your problems and so that you can decide whether or not you feel comfortable working with them. During the session, the Practitioner may tap on your meridians (located on the face, collarbone, hands, under arm and top of head) or ask you to tap as you repeat certain words and phrases. You may be asked to roll your eyes, hum and count but don't worry - this is purely to get your brain in gear!

What will I feel?

Everyone experiences different signs and sensations when using EFT. Some of these sensations are tightness or tingling in the body, feeling light-headed, warm, emotional or just feeling very relaxed are others. None of these are harmful it's just your energy moving around.

Can anyone use it?

Despite the amazing results you can achieve through EFT for a wide variety of psychological and physiological problems, EFT is a complementary therapy and should be applied responsibly. Don't view it as a remedy or a substitute for medical treatment in the case of acute problems.

Feldenkrais Method

What is it?

The Feldenkrais Method was developed by a Russian doctor, Dr Moshe Feldenkrais in the 1940's. It is a preventative therapy rather than a treatment and is similar in its approach to the Alexander Technique. It uses movement and awareness to improve flexibility and functioning of the body. Dr Feldenkrais believed that awareness is developed through experience and developed methods using movement to re-educate the body and to help to break down established patterns of behaviour.

Body awareness - posture, movement and spatial orientation - is the main key to the Feldenkrais Method. By becoming more conscious of how we move, areas that are less flexible and formed habitual patterns, then this creates an awareness that can be used to initiate change in how we choose to use our bodies. By repeated attention to how we move and by practising exercises to counter old patterns, the brain's signals to the body can be modified, becoming a new, 'chosen' way of moving. This can develop into a greater ease of movement, an increase in vitality and well-being.

Feldenkrais Method sessions can either be on a one-to-one basis or in group work. It encourages clients to take responsibility for themselves and anyone can benefit from this method as it's purpose is to discover the potential for living effortlessly according to each individual's abilities. It is therefore suitable for any age and most conditions, including neurological, conditions, orthopaedic problems, chronic and acute pain.

Feng Shui

What is it?

The history of the development of feng shui can be traced back for more than five thousand years. Feng shui has grown and adapted with the changing needs, desires and circumstances of humanity from both rural to urban environments.

The science originated in rural China when farmers studied their landscape, seasons, weather and many other factors to try to understand the environment that they lived in. They learned how the rivers changed course and their rates of flow, when the sun was high or low and the quality of its heat and which areas of land were saturated, fertile or parched and why.

Noticing the timing and quality of how the different energies all flowed together was complicated and scientific. It involved learning what the heavens and earth were doing and how the humans could successfully fit into the patterns. Their finely tuned expertise was purely observational, practical and common sense. This knowledge helped them to build their homes in the best positions, facing the most beneficial directions. They grew their crops in locations where they were most likely to have high yields. They survived well in their very harsh environments, building successful communities and prospering. Cities grew where the energies of meandering rivers, deep estuaries, protective mountains and flat lands combined in the most productive ways.

The Imperial rulers of China became interested in feng shui as they realised that it was a powerful science. Men that were skilled in the many styles of feng shui including Ba Chop, Sam Hap, Sam Yuan and Yuen Hom methods became Feng Shui Masters who served their Imperial ruler. These highly skills Masters protected their empire by choosing the best land for the ruler's palace, the best burial sites for their ancestry and the most opportune times for their ruler to act in order to succeed. This ensured that the ruler continued to reign powerfully and that he kept control and protected his people.

In the modern societies of today the focus it on living and working in crowded, urban environments where the pace of life is quick. How do we know if our environments are beneficial to us or whether we are being exhausted or harmed by their effects?

Form School

The shapes within our environment affect the way chi or lifeforce energy behaves. In analysing the form of your surroundings a skilled feng shui practitioner will be able to apply ancient principles concerning earth dragons and water dragons to interpret the modern urban or rural features of a property. For instance, a road is considered a type of 'river' and an aerial view of a neighbourhood can give some interesting insights into the fortunes of its inhabitants. Form accounts for 60% of the influences on a property.

At a micro level, the way chi flows through the interior of a property is also considered part of Form School theory. Good form is always prioritised.

Compass School

A building is like a human body. It has a 'mouth' (the door), eyes (windows), heart (often the kitchen) and a spine (the back). It also has a constitutional footprint, which is determined by the Ba Chop method and the relationship between the orientation of the building and the main front door.

The influence of time on a building is likened to it's 'acute' state, and this is where Flying Star comes in. Flying (as in moving over time) Stars are calculated to reveal the cosmic conditions affecting the building during a certain period of time. We are currently in the 8 fate, the cusp of which in Yuen Hom theory began in 1996 and in the Sam Yuan styles began in 1994. Within each year and month further refinements can be made to the calculations.

Geopathic Stress Detection

The assessment of underground waterways, energy courses and grave site selection is part of Yin Feng Shui and there are only a handful of truly skilled practitioners in the world. In certain situations Feng Shui remedies are far more effective once a premises the geopathic stress has been dealt with. Geopathic stress is a disturbance in the natural resonance of the earth's natural radiation (7.5 – 8 Hz) which causes a resonance in a building which is uncomfortably high for the human being to handle. It can cause insomnia, irritability, fatigue, and in some cases severe illness. Gypsies rarely suffer from cancer, as their nomadic lifestyle means they are never exposed to any harmful radiations coming from the earth.

Many practitioners can dowse for Negative or 'black' streams and locate the Positive or 'white' streams, in order to advise on placement of beds and desks, so that occupants are not subjected to geopathic stress. Geopathic stress neutralisers can also be purchased.

Space Clearing

Special herbs and resins are burned in a ceremonial and focussed way to cleanse the property of 'predecessor chi', stagnant energy and negative atmospheres. This is especially recommended in old homes or premises that have been lying empty or have witnessed divorces or deaths. It is also ideal to space clear a home before you move in.

Horoscope

An often overlooked area of Feng Shui is how an individual's birthdate relates to the property they inhabit, and how their Ba Zi (Four Pillars) horoscope may be impacting them at the time of their consultation. Knowledge of this very accurate astrology certainly helps a feng shui practitioner to make more informed recommendations to help their client.

Flower Essences

Since long before conventional medicine was developed, flowers have given us cause for wonder and been used for healing.

Our modern understanding and use of Flower Essences (or Flower Remedies) began with Dr Edward Bach in the early part of the 20th century. He was a successful Harley Street Doctor and Homeopath who felt his patients needed something more subtle to heal the emotional issues that underlay their symptoms. He identified 37 flowers and 1 other natural product (Rock Water) that he found had profound emotionally healing effects for his patients.

Since the latter part of the last century there has been a blossoming of this healing modality with many ranges now being made and used all over the world.

'Flower Essences' has become a generic term to include any vibrational essence. These include Gem and Mineral Essences, Animal Essences, Sound and music Essences, Environmental Essences, Colour

Essences, Angel and Divinity Essences and many others.

Theory and philosophy

Essences are energy medicine, they support our healing by helping us resolve emotional, mental and etheric patterns held in our energy fields. These are the scars developed from negative experiences and traumas over the courses of our lives. Some of these historic patterns may be with us all the time, creating underlying feelings from day to day; anxiety, suspicion, fear, sadness, shyness, anger etc, other patterns may get triggered in particular situations.

When a pattern is active we might experience emotional disturbance, or mental stress or habitual physical tensions. As well as being unhelpful in life, this can get in the way of our body's own healing process and lead to all sorts of physical symptoms.

According to modern physics, matter and energy are two sides of the same coin - $E=Mc^2$. Complex systems of matter, such as living things, have more complex energy structures. When two energy fields meet, there is an exchange of information. When we are in the presence of a flower (or other natural energy signature) our system is informed by it's energy and we can assimilate the particular information that our system needs for it's healing.

You may know from experience how healing it feels just being in a garden full of flowers, or in a pristine natural environment. Why do we give flowers to people recovering from illness or suffering bereavement?

Essences are the result of transferring the healing patterns of energy from natural realms into a liquid medium. This is accomplished by placing healthy flowers (or gems etc), at the peak of their perfection into a crystal bowl of pure water that is left to potentise in the sun. The resulting infusion is preserved (usually in alcohol or brine) and now carries the healing vibration from the flower.

Individual flowers and their essences have characteristics which, when we match them to our own mental and emotional state, can have a profound healing effect.

Healing

What is it?

I doubt there can be a therapy as ancient as the art of healing, although it may not have been called thus in the beginning of mankind. The very first use of the power of healing may have been by a mother wanting to comfort a hurt child and placing her hands over a bruise, or kissing the child better. Without perhaps being aware of it, this mother is transmitting a healing energy as her love goes to the child.

Nowadays, healing comes in many different forms and names and although the underlying principles may be similar, the beliefs about what makes the healing possible are many. Some people would call it a gift from God, others will claim to be helped by spirit guides, whilst others will have a much more pragmatic approach and talk about energy fields. Most healers believe that they are channeling an energy which exists all around us. This energy helps repair and re-establish balance in the aura around a person and, through that, affect changes at a physiological or psychological level as well as work at a spiritual level. The healing of one person by another can be done either from a distance or by the laying-on of hands.

Although the many forms of healing have been derided by the orthodox medical establishment for far too long, many people have benefited from receiving healing. It is only very recently that some people in the medical world have started to accept that healing can be beneficial, to the extent that healers can now be found in some hospitals and clinics.

During healing, you will most probably be asked to sit upright or to lie down, relax and close your eyes whilst the healer passes his or her hands over you, usually a few centimetres away from your body. You may experience a sensation or warmth and energy through you and become very relaxed indeed. You may also feel energised. Some people begin to feel better almost immediately whilst others may not feel any benefit for days or weeks, and then not always in the ways in which it was expected.

Although it is hoped that any physical symptoms can be "cured" as a result of the exchange of energy, sometime the healing will happen by first creating within the patient a greater understanding of what they are going through and of the steps they may need to take to help themselves.

Hellerwork

What is it?

Joseph Heller started Hellerwork in the late 1970's. Heller had originally trained with Ida Rolf and became president of the Rolf Institute in 1975; however, he wanted to explore the mind/body connection further and left to start his own school.

Hellerwork has three basic concepts:

Bodywork - deep tissue massage that unblocks the body
Movement Education - to correct postural alignment
Verbal Dialogue - to assess emotional holding patterns.

Hellerworkers believe that not only is memory held in the brain, but also in the muscles and tissues of the body - therefore by changing someone's body on a structural level, you will affect their being on an emotional level and vice versa. The massage used concentrates on the body's fascia (the connective tissue that contains and links the muscles and muscle fibres, as well as forms the tendons and ligaments of the body) the movement education works on the principle that the body must be straight and evenly balanced, with the line of gravitational force running down the centre. Specific exercises are given to remedy any problems. Verbal dialogue is a psychotherapeutic technique that attempts to identify and remedy the cause of any troublesome state of mind, in order to release areas of the body that may be affected.

What to expect:

Hellerwork has a rigid structure of eleven sessions lasting 90 minutes each. The first session will include a detailed history, and a study of how you walk, sit and stand. Before and after photographs may also be taken. Further sessions will be divided into three main groups targeting certain areas - the Superficial section, the Core section and the Integrative section. After the eleven sessions are completed, advice will be given on exercises to do at home, and follow-up sessions will be recommended after any physical or emotional trauma.

Herbal medicine

What is it?

As a form of treatment that is said to be as old as mankind itself, it is interesting to notice that this most ancient form of medicine is coming back to challenge the most sophisticated system of medicine in the world's history. Today, the World Health Organisation estimates that, worldwide, herbal medicine is three to four times more commonly practised than conventional medicine.

It can be said that the origins of modern medicine, with its heavy reliance on drug prescription to treat specific diseases, lie in herbal medicine. Some of the best modern drugs are purified products of herbs, and in worldwide use.

Primitive tribes still use their traditional knowledge of plants and their healing properties and, in early civilisations, food and medicine were closely linked together, as many plants were eaten for their health-giving properties.

Much of Britain's knowledge about the use of herbs can be traced back to ancient Egypt where the priests kept that knowledge. A papyrus from the city of Thebes dating back from 1500 BC lists hundreds of medicinal herbs, including many that are still in use today.

The ancient Greeks and Romans also were practitioner of herbal medicine and much of their knowledge has been passed on as their armies conquered the world and military doctors took the plants and their uses with them. Two more cultures which have always relied very heavily on herbal medicine are the Chinese and the Indians and, to this day, China herbs play a vital part in health care.

In Britain, from the Dark Ages well into medieval times, herbals were painstakingly hand-copied in the monasteries, each of which had its own physic garden for growing herbs to treat both monks and local people. In rural areas, particularly in the west and Wales, the Druids are believed to have had an oral tradition of herbal medicine, mixing medicine with mysticism and rituals.

The crucial difference between medical herbalists and today's orthodox doctor is, firstly, that the herbalist looks at the patient as a whole, while conventional doctors look for symptoms which enable them to diagnose and treat diseases. They see the person as the carrier of a disease, whilst the herbalist regards the patient as a diseased person, requiring a holistic treatment. Secondly, the medical herbalist is using whole plants or plant products containing active constituents, while doctors use these constituents in refined and isolated forms or synthetics.

As medical herbalists have become more scientifically minded in their research, so a new word has been coined to described their work: phytotherapy, from the Greek words phyton, meaning 'plant', and therapeuein, 'to take care of, to heal'.

A medical herbalist will treat the patient as an individual , with individual weaknesses and needs. He/She is likely to enquire about lifestyle, diet, stresses and look for any imbalance and disharmony, seeking the cause of the illness. Each treatment is tailored to specific and varying requirements.

Holographic Repatterning

What is it?

Holographic repatterning is based on the principle of resonance. Founder Chloe Faith Wordsworth worked as a complementary healer for 30 years, she studied and practiced different types of healing but found that what worked for one person did not necessarily work for another. She synthesized her training and experience in complementary therapies with her knowledge of psychology and physics to come up with the concept of HR. Chloe compares a human being to a hologram - a holographic plate can accommodate millions of images; one only has to change the angle of the light to see a different picture. She describes HR as 'a method to identify and transform non-coherent frequencies that cause us to resonate with life depleting patterns that are preventing us from resonating with life-enhancing patterns.'

The HR practitioner believes that no matter how a problem manifests itself it could be physical pain or emotional disfunction, the underlying issue has to be identified and shifted. This is commonly referred to as an energy block - HR practitioners see themselves as facilitators to rid us of these blocks. In HR, a pattern is identified through discussion and a technique learned from kinesiology - a method of taping into body intelligence developed by an American chiropractor called muscle checking. The principle is biofeedback, meaning that the body and mind respond at a purely unconscious level.

What to expect

A session can last up to two hours, and there is no way of saying how many sessions it takes to release limiting thought processes - for some a one off is all it will take, whilst for others a few sessions are required. The client is required to lie prone on a mat or bed and is asked to relax, once the client gives the practitioner permission to work on them an energy transaction will begin. The practitioner tunes into and accesses information through a muscle check, using the client's arm as an indicator in the process. The belief in HR is that various 'healing modalities' like movement, sound, colour and other energetic objects (such as crystals) can be applied to effect an improvement in the clients condition. The HR practitioner believes that the therapy can help with chronic poor health, unhappy relationships, failure, low confidence, depression and other life-depleting responses by allowing the client to identify and transform patterns that have held them in limitation and pain, it enables the client to find out which self-healing modalities would work best for them.

Holographic Repatterning can be used as a treatment on its own, or to support other healing systems. It can be done as a self-help treatment, practiced on family and friends, or studied in order to attain professional certified status.

Homoeopathy

What is it Homoeopathy?

Homoeopathy is a system of prescribing which uses plants, minerals, and some animal remedies, prescribed on the principle that "Like cures like". This is called the simile principle. The word "homoeopathy" is derived from the Greek words "homoios" meaning like or similar, and "pathos" meaning suffering.

" Let like be cured by like"

This exploits the property of some medicinal substances to stimulate the natural healing energy of the individual. The activity of this healing process is demonstrated by the symptoms of an illness, and a remedy is chosen which has been found when taken by healthy volunteers to cause symptoms similar to that illness.

This system of therapeutics was discovered by Hahnemann at the end of the eighteenth century. He found that cinchona bark, which was used to treat swamp fever (now known as malaria), when taken by him produced the same symptoms as the disease. Here was a strange phenomenon, a remedy which was an effective treatment for a disease inducing the symptoms of that disease when given to a healthy person. He decided to experiment further. He took further doses himself, and gave some to his family.

He found in every case that symptoms of swamp fever occurred on taking the cinchona bark, which stopped on ceasing to take it.

He now began to determine and record the effect of a large number of substances on the human body. He gathered together a band of helpers to whom he gave remedies, interrogating them daily on sensations experienced .He called this a proving. He was thus able to produce a materia medica consisting of symptoms produced in healthy volunteers. This materia medica represented a vast collection of very accurate observations. These pictures, when matched with the symptoms of a sick person, enabled him to identify the remedy which would cure the patient. He found when actually treating patients that a small material dose of the substance would produce an aggravation of symptoms before it cured. He then started to dilute the remedies, and vigorously shaking them (succussing) between dilutions. This produced a cure without the aggravation. He also found that a remedy so treated was more powerful as a curative, and so he called the process potensisation.

Homoeopathy is still based on this principle when used today, 200 years later then Hahnemann's time. It is very different from conventional medicine and is frequently misunderstood and denigrated . In conventional medicine we are taught to think in terms of disease and pathological states, changes from the normal physiological state wrought by outside factors such as infection trauma and stress, and also conditions arising from allergy or even autoimmunity. In order to treat such disease states we try to make a diagnosis based on symptoms and physical signs. This may enable us to find a cause for which there is a specific treatment or failing this, to treat the patient's complaints by symptomatic measures. Although there has been an increasing emphasis on treating the patient as a whole, medicine is in actual fact becoming increasingly fragmented and specialised, and there are few treatments which cure the patient as a whole.

If we look more closely at the patient, we find that although symptoms of a disease fall into a variety of categories which are more or less well defined, there are also other symptoms present. These vary from case to case, and are unique to that person. Thus no one case, even of a well defined disease like chickenpox, or pneumonia, exactly resembles another, any more than two individuals are ever absolutely identical. In other words the symptoms and signs of the disease are modified by the reaction of the patient.

The basis of homoeopathy is that the most successful remedy for any given occasion will be the one whose symptomatology presents the clearest and closest resemblance to the symptom complex of the sick person in question.

That is: let like be treated by like. Examples of this are as follows:-

The effects of peeling an onion are very similar to the symptoms of a cold or hay fever, and the remedy prepared from onion is used to treat colds and hay fever where the symptoms are similar.

The symptoms and signs of arsenic poisoning are very similar to those of certain cases of gastro-enteritis, and the remedy arsenicum album is used to treat these cases, with success.

So the first and fundamental principle of homoe-opathy is the selection and use of a similar remedy.

The second and more controversial issue is the use of remedies in apparently very small quantities. This in itself is not homoeopathy but a refining of the basic method worked out by Hahnemann. Recent research has indicated that during potentisation an imprint of the molecular structure of the remedy is left in the liquid ,and this is therapeutically active.

Further research has shown that homoeopathic remedies are more successful than placebo and in some cases than conventional treatment in certain illnesses. It is believed that the natural healing pro-cess of the organism is stimulated by the remedy.

In spite of the general scepticism of many con-ventional medical practitioners homoeopathy works and has a place in modern therapeutics. It is prescribable on the NHS, and has been used by the Royal Family for many years.

Homoeopathic treatment can aid recovery in many conditions where a medical practitioner might wish to avoid the use of allopathic medicines. Since it stimulates the natural healing process there is less likelihood of recurrence of the condition, and homoeopathic treatment leads to an improvement in general health. There are applications for the use of homoeopathy in some conditions which are difficult to treat by conventional means. Remedies may afford relief to sufferers who find side effects of some drugs too unpleasant. Homoeopathic remedies can be used together with allopathic drugs and other conventional treatment quite safely and effectively, they are without side effects and can be used in pregnancy, for young infants, and the elderly; they are inexpensive and treatment is cost-effective.

Homoeopathy is indicated in the treatment of many conditions:

in the initial treatment of acute infections, of the upper and lower respiratory tract, and skin.

for chronic conditions such as skin disease, arthritis, postviral fatigue.

for recurrent conditions-upper respiratory tract infections, glue ear, rhinitis, bronchitis, cystitis, vaginitis.

in the treatment of hormone related diseases-PMT, endometriosis, and menopausal problems.

for psychosomatic problems, stress related illnesses, including headaches, migraine, backache and muscular tension.

for allergies
for depression and anxiety
Hopi Ear Candles

What are Hopi Ear Candles?

Hopi ear candles are named after the Native American tribe who first introduced this gentle therapy to the West.

The Hopi nation is renowned for their extensive knowledge of healing and their spiritual lifestyle. The translation of the word Hopi means "peaceful ones".

Ear candles are used widely throughout North America and Asia and although the current treatment has come to us from the Hopi tribe, the use of ear candles to treat ear problems has been known for centuries, having been used by the Egyptians, Romans and Greeks.

What is a Hopi Ear Candle?

Ear candles are an ancient, mild and natural therapy and have been used by the Native American Indian for many years.

The Hopi candle is not a candle as such, but a hollow tube made out of cotton flax. To stiffen the flax, they are impregnated with extract of honey and herb oils (in particular chamomile, sage and St Johns wort), the healing properties of which have been known to the Hopi tribe for hundreds of years. The making of the candles is a complex process and all genuine Hopi candles are made in the traditional manner.

The Treatment

The treatment is very gentle and relaxing and may take up to an hour, depending on the condition being treated.

The candle is placed over the ear orifice and ignited. It is only allowed to burn to within 4 inches of the end of the candle. As it burns it produces a gentle local heat. The warm air combined with the oil and herbs soften the wax and draw it into the base of the candle. The candle is then removed and the ear and surrounding area is then massaged. The treatment is repeated on the other ear and then a complete facial massage is carried out, paying particular attention to the sinus areas.

What Conditions can Ear Candles Help?

Ear candles can help with the treatment of sinusitis, rhinitis, earwax, earache and irritation of the ears including tinnitus. It is also suitable for the treatment of headaches and migraines. It is not suitable for those with perforated eardrums, where grommets are in place or those who may have an allergy to the ingredients. It is a safe and gentle treatment for children.

The number of treatments depends on how long the candle takes to burn down. Each treatment takes approximately 45 - 60 minutes and is very relaxing. It is advisable to put a few drops of warm olive oil in each ear for three days before treatment as this will help to soften the wax which will make it easier to remove. On the day of the treatment, you will be advised to remove all makeup and earrings

Hypnotherapy

What is it?

Hypnotherapy has nothing to do with what can be seen on stage where performers try to manipulate people into acting in silly ways. Unfortunately, much of the public knowledge of hypnosis is based on such shows which very often leads to a fear of hypnosis and a reluctance on the part of many people to seek for the help that hypnotherapy can give.

Somewhere between wakefulness and sleep is the state of consciousness that hypnotherapists use. That trance like state is similar to the one that occurs spontaneously in sleepwalking or daydreaming. Most people will experience hypnosis as a state in which they become more aware of their inner being, their emotions and state of mind so as to make it possible to work and transform those emotions and states which may have become a problem. You will not lose consciousness or awareness, but become able to gain a different perspective on what has been troubling you.

Most people talk and act as if the conscious mind is the prime mover behind our behaviour and regard the unconscious mind as something vague, that they are not really aware of. In fact, the unconscious mind is always working, monitoring and affecting all the physical and psychological functions of the mind and the body, from blood pressure and hormone levels to states of hunger and fatigue, even when we are asleep. The sum of what we have learned and experienced is also stored within the unconscious mind, and our memory holds far more than we can usually remember at a conscious level

Through accessing that unconscious mind, hypnotherapy can help you learn how to react differently to certain situations and help you to understand better the development mechanism of your mind. For example, if you have to prepare for an exam and feel nervous about it, you can learn how to access and strengthen your ability to relax and apply that to the situation of passing an exam. Once you know how to do that, then it becomes easier to "decide" how you would like to feel and react in a given situation.

It also is possible with hypnotherapy to access memories and past events which are still having a detrimental impact on the present. By understanding better what happened and how patterns of behaviour and feelings were created, then it becomes possible to transform how those memories affect us in our life. You can't erase and forget the past, but you can learn to feel differently about it.

What will happen?

Really, that will depend on what is troubling you. A good therapist will try to help you understand what is the root cause of your problem and how to transform your response to it.

Remember that you already have within yourself the answers to the problem, even if you are not aware of that at a conscious level. No matter how good he/she is, the therapist cannot just give you the answers that you seek as he/she cannot know what is the best solution for you. He/she can only help you to find those answers within yourself and help you draw on your existing resources to transform your emotional difficulties. The therapist will help you access and utilise those resources so that you may learn how to make better use of them.

What is it best for?

Hypnotherapy is particularly useful in helping people to deal with stress and anxiety related conditions such as panic attacks, phobias, insomnia and other emotional problems like depression, lack of confidence and self esteem, etc.

It can also be of help with problems such as irritable bowel syndrome, migraine, skin problems, ulcers, asthma and high blood pressure. It can be of great help in the management of chronic pain.

Hypnotherapy can also help you change unwelcome habits such as smoking and nail-biting, and deal with problems relating to food and body image. This is achieved by finding out what the real problem is and finding better, more positive ways to meet your needs.

Indian Head Massage (IHM)

What is it?

Indian Head Massage is a treatment based on old Ayurvedic techniques involving work on the upper back, shoulders, neck, scalp and face. A variety of massage movements are used to relieve accumulated tension, stimulate circulation and restore joint movement. IHM is also used to aid the condition and health of the hair, particularly when combined with the use of natural organic oils.

Indian Head Massage is used by practitioners to help reduce stress and fatigue, increase mental clarity, and relax and rejuvenate the receiver. A treatment will last between 20 minutes to one hour.

Iridology

What is it?

Iridology was developed in Hungary in the 19th Century and involves the study of the Iris of the eye (the coloured sector) and the Pupil, using microscopic analysis of the surface structures to determine the health of the whole body. Genetic strengths and weaknesses, levels of inflammation and toxicity, the efficiency of the eliminative organs all build up a picture of both current health status and predispositions. An Iridologist may use a specialist camera to take pictures of a client's iris, or simply examine them with an ophthalmoscope and will not claim to diagnose an actual disease with these methods, but to identify weaknesses in the body.

Iridology is a safe, non-invasive and inexpensive method of analysis that can be integrated into both orthodox and complementary medicine. Medical research in several European countries and Russia in particular has established greater acceptance of Iridology. In Russia, a trial involving 800,000 patients found Iridology to be 85% accurate in diagnosis; in South Korea clinical trials by the government found that on average Iridology was 78.2% accurate but with an impressive 90.2% accuracy in the diagnosis of digestive system disorders. By contrast, orthodox medicine considers other diagnostic techniques as reliable if they are accurate within a range of 30 - 40%.

Iridology has much to offer medicine. It is already taught to medical students in certain European universities. In the USA, a professorship has recently been conferred on a Fellow of The Guild of Naturopathic Iridology by a leading medical teaching university. His role there is to instigate the teaching of Iridology in particular plus other forms of complementary medicine. Gradually Iridology will become an integrated diagnostic method.

The human iris and pupil - the eye- is one of the most intricate structures in nature and is one of the most visible parts. Its thousands of nerve endings are connected to the brain via the hypothalamus, giving readouts on conditions in all organs and systems of the body. The iris provides accurate information about our constitutional type, helping patients to understand their strengths and weaknesses, thereby enabling them to become more personally aware of what they can do to help themselves in both the short and long-term. As bodily tissues become inflamed or congested, the iris registers the processes, enabling the Iridologist to determine the root cause of current disorders. For example, a toxic digestive system may be responsible for seemingly unrelated problems such as migraines, skin disorders or joint problems

A few minutes focused observation of the eyes will point you in the right direction, saving a great deal of time, energy, guesswork and frustration. By establishing the root cause of disorders, an appropriately trained and qualified Iridologist can advise the most effective forms of therapy that will attain the best results for the individual - a truly wholistic approach. Members of The Guild of Naturopathic Iridology are qualified not only in Iridology but also in at least one other therapeutic science e.g. herbal medicine, homoeopathy, orthodox medicine, nutrition, naturopathy.

Johrei

What is it?

Johrei is a Japanese therapy started in the early 20th century. Described as more of a way of life than a therapy, Johrei aims to eliminate toxins from the body through touch, and promotes a more natural way of living.

A treatment lasts between 60 and 90 minutes, and is conducted with the client fully clothed and sat on the floor or a futon. The therapist will ask questions about physical and mental health, he or she will then hold their hands over your body to channel healing energy, areas of toxic build up are found using gentle pressure and then channeled to the kidneys, which flush out any toxins.

Practitioners claim that Johrei boosts the body's immune system by eliminating toxins and encouraging the body to heal itself. The treatment is also beneficial for stress related conditions, allergies and chronic pain. Clients are encouraged to devote time to their health requirements, and initially 2 or 3 treatments a week may be recommended.

Johrei is given on a one-to-one basis by a qualified therapist, although workshops are available to encourage people to study the method and use it on family and friends.

Kahuna Bodywork (or Hawaiian Massage, Lomi Lomi)

What is it?

Kahuna bodywork is a healing art originating in Hawaii. There are different forms and until recently, Kahuna bodywork was only passed down through oral tradition from one generation in a family to the next.

The word Kahuna has many meanings, one definition is "Spiritual keeper of knowledge, priest or shaman and masters of the art".

Traditionally, Kahuna bodywork was carried out on three consecutive days and often received on special ceremonial days by Hawaiian royalty. Each day was aimed at restoring balance and harmony to the client, the first being the physical level, the second day relating to the emotional self and the last day working at the 'bone level' which is seen as an opportunity for new growth and spiritual aspects. Today, the average session lasts approximately two hours.

Kahuna bodywork is a deep and rhythmical massage. The rhythm is very relaxing and works gently but deeply into the muscles using continuous flowing strokes. The energy comes from the use of this rhythm and movement, creating a continuous ebb and flow between the practitioner and the client. The practitioner uses the forearm, fingers, heel and palm of the hand in long, flowing movements over the body that bring fresh oxygen to every cell. Various massage techniques are used to relax the muscles, increase circulation and break down adhesions and to increase the vibrational rate of the cells of the body. Acupressure points may also be used, plus warm stone therapy, breathing techniques, chanting, music, visualisations, herbs and aromas depending on the lineage of the practitioner.

A main principle of Kahuna bodywork is to encourage clients to know themselves better by inwardly listening to their own bodies and experiences and aims to help clients accept their own body and love themselves. Whilst the technique is an important part of the massage and associated healing, the practitioner works in harmony with the client with love and compassion to connect to one's own self-love which is believed to strengthen the ability to recognise the beauty in our life and surroundings. One of the tenets of Kahuna bodywork is everything seeks harmony and everything seeks love.

Kanpo

What is it?

Herbal medicine has been practiced in Japan for many centuries. It has benefited from influences from all over Asia, which were synthesised with the ancient native Japanese medicine and evolved into what is now known as Kanpo. Kanpo is a practical form of herbal medicine based on a wealth of experience and modern clinical research. It is a holistic form of therapy as many factors about the individual are considered when determining which herbs to give. It is widely used in Japan today.

Kanpo treatment is said to support the body's own natural healing mechanisms. Diagnosis involves taking a case history and carefully examining the patient's tongue, abdomen and pulse - from an Oriental medical perspective. A herbal formula is then selected which the practitioner feels reflects the patient needs, as treatment progresses and the patient's condition alters, a different formula will be selected. Originally crude herbs were given to the patient to prepare, but recently herbal extracts are most often given. These come in an extract or granule form and are easy and convenient to take. They are strictly quality controlled and Good Manufacturing Practice (GMP) is used at every stage from growing to harvesting, and preparing the formulae. These formulae do not rely upon rare species, or the ill treatment of animals. In Japan, Kanpo is regulated by the Japanese Government. All Kanpo medicines are continually being assessed with regards to both safety and efficiency, to ensure their position in the modern context of Japanese primary healthcare. The Journal of the Royal Society of Medicine recently reported on a UK safety study of Kanpo medicine. The six-year study took place in a London NHS practice and results, based on blood analysis, showed no adverse effects on patients treated with Kanpo medicine.

Kanpo is used to treat a wide range of conditions, both acute and chronic. It is traditionally used to treat digestive, cardiovascular, respiratory, urinary, reproductive system and skin disorders. In recent times the structure and pattern of diseases has altered with an increase in immune system disorders and stress related conditions - Kanpo is being used to treat these also. It is also said to be of benefit as an adjunct to western medical treatment, softening the adverse reactions. Kanpo can be used in addition to other therapies, as well as complementing treatment from a doctor.

Kinesiology

What is it?

The word 'kinesiology' comes from the Greek work kineses, which means motion. In the medical sciences it is the name given to the study of muscles and the movement of the body. 'Applied Kinesiology' was the name given by its inventor, Dr George Goodheart, to the system of applying muscle testing diagnostically and therapeutically to different aspects of health care. Today Applied Kinesiology refers only to the parent system, as taught by the International College of Applied Kinesiology. As a number of different branches have evolved, the term Kinesiology has come to be accepted as a general term for all of these systems.

Kinesiology is a system of diagnosis and treatment that asks the body what it wants by combining muscle testing with the principles of Chinese medicine, to assess energy and body function, using a range of gentle yet powerful techniques. Muscle testing is the principal method of assessment used in Kinesiology, and it is the use of muscle testing that distinguishes it from other therapies. There are a number of different ways of using muscle testing in assessment - as a series of specific muscles tests, to find out how well the body is functioning in all aspects - structural, chemical and emotional, and with an indicator muscle test, which uses a single muscle to get a non-verbal response to a stimulus. All branches of Kinesiology use both methods, and some branches make greater use of the indicator muscle test.

The Kinesiology Federation gives the following definition:

'Kinesiology, literally the study of body movement, is a holistic approach to balancing the movement and interaction of a person's energy systems. Gentle assessment of muscle response monitors those areas where blocks and imbalances are impairing physical, emotional or energetic well -being. The same method can identify factors that may be contributing to such imbalances. The body's natural healing responses are stimulated by attention to reflex and acupressure points, and by use of specific body movements and nutritional support. These can lead to increased physical and mental, emotional and spiritual well-being.'

What to expect

Almost all Kinesiologists will give a session lasting one hour or longer. Much of the first session will be spent in gathering information, in order that the practitioner can built up a picture of the balance of your structural, nutritional and emotional state. The Kinesiologist will pay attention to any specific symptoms you may have, but all aspects will by covered, as it is a holistic treatment. At the end of the first session, the practitioner will be able to give you a summary of the main areas of imbalance that your body has shown. You may also be told about the corrections you have been given. You may be advised to attend weekly for three to four sessions, and then at less frequent intervals.

Life-coaching

What is it?

Life-coaching is a means of bridging the gap between where you are now and where you want to be. It often involves clarifying those two first.

Life-coaching works through a dynamic partnership focussed entirely on the client and the client's agenda. Our lives have become so complex, opportunities so plentiful, that exploring what's important to us as individuals and our own unique situation is the quickest and often the only way to know exactly what to change and how to change it. And to identify and move beyond those things that are holding us back from the lives we really want.

In life-coaching, people experience significant shifts in their lives. They become clearer on who they are and what they need in their lives to be fulfilled. Living the live that's truly right for them, it all becomes easier, more joyful. They also get to do, be or have more of what they want or need in every conceivable area. Better than this, they do so more quickly and easily, with more enjoyment and far less stress. They go from being driven by need to inspired by their goals or life. And they create the conditions to easily sustain this easier, happier way of living.

Clarity

Coaching often starts by exploring what the person really wants. Even when people believe they know this, greater clarity and self-awareness emerge through coaching. And sometimes, people discover different aspirations, ones that make them want to leap out of bed each morning.

The focus of coaching and the skills and objectivity of our coach enable us to know ourselves more fully than ever before. And, rather like a sports coach watching an athlete, a trained listener hears and reflects back to us subtle and fleeting clues to our unique motivations, like a change in voice tone or energy level.

Growth

What we learn about ourselves through coaching will include our potential and gifts, but also anything we may have previously avoided. A priceless benefit of having a coach is that an independent professional with your best interests at heart will tell you necessary truths when others won't - and tell it within a context of genuine praise and belief in you and your ability to change that makes it easier to hear.

As coaching proceeds clients come to feel more and more comfortable in their lives. However, like anything that stretches you, coaching won't always feel comfortable. Your coach will challenge you and ask more of you than you would of yourself. You needn't accept all your coach's requests but once you choose to commit to something, your coach will hold you to it - and to being the best you can be. As coaching progresses, you will know from your actions that you are indeed capable of more.

You'll make choices and step outside your comfort zone. But you will do so far more easily than you otherwise would and witness your comfort zone rapidly expand. Any temporary discomfort is vastly outweighed by the delight of leaping over hurdles you wouldn't even have approached before. And of living a life that really suits you.

Holistic and sustainable

When we know what we really want for ourselves, we have more energy, focus and direction. Regular coaching builds momentum, sustains inspiration and enables people to be consistently at their best. Clients mobilize more effective resources and discover the quickest, easiest and most enjoyable way forward.

All coaching is holistic - no goal is allowed to become more important than the person. Coaching often includes building or fine-tuning an environment and support systems so that they provide the structure that ensures your on-going ease, sparkle and success. It may involve streamlining, to reclaim energy drained off in secondary activities. And it frequently leads to better resources, be they cutting edge tools for personal development, connections or whatever else will be most useful at that time.

What does life-coaching cover?

Any or all aspects of your life. Some people come for specific issues (such as health, relationships, finances or a transition) or projects (like creating a new life or developing a seminar program). Some come to enjoy more what they've already got, to fine-tune some aspects of their life or for self-development. Others are drawn to coaching by a general dissatisfaction or a sense that something could be better. And some create more space for themselves and for spontaneous, joyous action by cutting back on their commitments.

What's coaching like?

Coaching sessions are friendly, relaxed but focussed and amazingly powerful on many levels. Most coaching takes place through regular, pre-arranged telephone sessions. Email coaching can also be very effective and clients benefit from both, with email coaching between calls.

Manual Lymphatic Drainage (MLD)

What is it?

Manual Lymph Drainage is an advanced form of massage that aims to stimulate the lymphatic system to remove congestion and stagnation from within the body, and so help it return to a healthy condition. Dr Emil Vodder, who was able to show that many chronic conditions could be alleviated with lymphatic drainage and massage techniques, developed it in the 1930's

A true therapist will be trained in a recognized method such as Vodder or Casley-Smith. The treatment will involve a consultation and a massage using gentle rhythmic pumping techniques. Follow up advice on diet and other ways to stimulate the lymph may also be given.

Symptoms that are said to respond well to MLD are a weakened immune system, chronic congestion (sinus etc), rheumatoid arthritis and the healing of wounds, burns and scars. MLD is also often incorporated into the treatment and control of Lymphoedema.

McTimoney Chiropractic

What is it?

McTimoney Chiropractic began in the 1950's when John McTimoney sought treatment from a chiropractor for a damaged arm. He was so impressed with his treatment that he decided to study the method, and quickly became a talented healer. He began to experiment with the technique, refining the movements and incorporating the whole body into a treatment - his school was established in 1972.

What to expect from a treatment

A McTimoney Chiropractor will always start a treatment by taking a full case history, with many questions on past accidents, falls, injuries and illnesses. The client is then asked to undress down to their underwear and the practitioner will examine by hand the bones and joints of the body to check for any imbalances - however subtle they may be. The method used for correcting and imbalance is called the toggle-recoil, which is used to change the tension surrounding a joint - it is not a forced movement but rather a rapid thrust followed by an immediate release. The treatment is relatively gentle to receive as it uses the natural elasticity of tendons to help relieve muscle tension.

Medau Movement

What is it?

Medau Movement is an approach to exercise that aims to bring about whole body natural movement. Emphasis is placed to using the body correctly, as posture and alignment are seen as vital in the maintenance of good health. Medau aims to improve awareness of the importance of the body's structure, and help to rectify imbalances through movement.

A Medau class should be challenging, enjoyable and fun, with varying types of music being played to complement the exercises being used. As well as whole body awareness being improved, Medau can also help to reduce stress levels. The exercises and movements used in a class are suitable for a wide age range.

Meditation

What is it?

Meditation is a safe and simple way to help you move towards balance and harmony and is often used as a path towards knowledge of the Self. It is a practice that is perhaps as old as mankind and can be used as an aid in dealing with stress and illnesses.

A state of meditation happens when your attention is focused upon the experience of the moment and is often reached by the use of techniques to calm the mind and body. There are several forms of meditation, most of which can be grouped into two basic approaches:

Focused or concentrative meditation
Mindfulness

Whilst the first brings a narrowing of the attention upon a particular subject such as an image, a mantra or other symbols, the second tends to be more like observing the flow of experiences and sensations without interfering with them. Some practices are a mix of those two approaches. Focused meditation can be likened to looking through a microscope, it helps us go deeper into the experience, whilst a state of mindfulness can be more like gazing through a window, noticing everything that passes and our own experiences in relation to what is being observed. Both approaches can be combined with great effects.

With the practice of meditation, you can learn how to relax and how to direct your attention for the purpose of exploring your Self and learning about your own emotional and mental responses. It is a useful tool in the quest for understanding, self knowledge and spiritual development. Meditation should only be taught by an experienced and knowledgeable teacher who will be able to guide you in your inner journey, thus helping you to understand better what you may encounter and how to work with it.

When in meditation, the mind is in a state of restful alertness whilst the body becomes more relaxed, thus allowing for a natural healing and harmonising to take place. The benefits of meditation can be found on three levels: physical, psychological and spiritual.

Physical benefits: It has been shown that the regular use of meditation can strengthen the immune system, making it better able to resist infections. Physiological problems that are stress related, or influenced by stress, can also be helped as the meditator learns to cope better and to respond more positively to the stressful situation

Psychological benefits: Meditation can help most people feel more relaxed and better able to cope with life's events. It can promote a more aware attitude, leading to a recognition of the choices one has in life. This can help the meditator to realise that life is not something that just happens to us, but something that is to be embraced and where the person has power.

Spiritual benefits: To tell someone what to believe is to take away their freedom. Meditation is a personal journey towards understanding and knowledge of Self and of the Source. It is an exploration that has the potential to reveal the secrets of life. Meditation will help you find your own answers... and many more questions.

Metabolic Typing

What is it?

Metabolic typing - the classic definition

In short, Metabolic Typing is "customised nutrition" based on the idea that there is no universal healthy diet to suit everyone.

Anyone can use Metabolic Typing find out exactly which foods are good for their health, and those that are not. You will find out about the supplements you need that will make you as healthy as you can be and not waste your money on those that could make you tired and sick.

Metabolic Typing is a process of evaluating the inter-relationship of the body's 3 main systems for the creation and maintenance of energy.

These are the Autonomic Nervous System, the Oxidative System and the Endocrine System.

It is the name given to the analysis of individual nutritional needs and biochemical individuality.

Metabolic Typing interprets and understands "body language", which is the body's means of communicating its physical, mental, emotional and behavioural characteristics, as well as its efficiency and homeostatic balance, through which, individual nutritional requirements may be understood and applied.

Metabolic typing is based on the understanding that although there are tens of thousands of biochemical reactions that take place in your body every day, they all fall under the control of only a few Fundamental Homeostatic Controls. The Healthexcel System of Metabolic Typing recognises 9 such control mechanisms and uses them to evaluate and determine each person's metabolic type. It is the inherited various strengths and weaknesses in these control mechanisms that define our biochemical individuality and makes each of us unique. Importantly, every food and every nutrient has very specific effects on these Fundamental Controls. For this reason, not knowing one's metabolic type makes it impossible to know which foods or nutrients are best for each person.

No adverse condition can exist without a metabolic imbalance in one or more of these systems. These metabolic imbalances are very common, and most people who are chronically unwell have at least one of them. Correcting them usually results in major improvements in health. Many chronic health problems can be expected to clear up when these imbalances are corrected. In fact, you must correct these imbalances to see many, if not most chronic conditions heal.

When a person is "balanced" metabolically, many disease symptoms subside because the body uses nutrients optimally. It is important to understand that metabolic typing does not address any specific conditions, using a "One Size Fits All" approach like allopathic nutrition.

This symptom/treatment method, therefore has no rational basis in seeking a common protocol for all people with a certain condition. Any success would be down to chance and could not be relied upon. Remember that if nutrition can help, it can also harm.

Metamorphic Technique

What is the Metamorphic Technique?

The Metamorphic Technique is a simple approach to self-healing and personal development. We all have great potential, but due to limiting beliefs that we hold about ourselves and our lives, we tend to get ourselves stuck in particular patterns that keep us from fully realising that potential. These patterns can show up in various ways - physical or mental illness, emotional problems, limiting attitudes or repeating patterns of behaviour. Beneath these external symptoms are corresponding patterns of energy. The Metamorphic Technique acts as a catalyst to this energy (also known as the life force), gently enabling you to transform your patterns and begin to move from who you are, to who you can be.

The Metamorphic practitioner uses a light touch on points known as the spinal reflexes in the feet, hands and head. At the same time, he or she remains detached from the achievement of specific results. This allows your energy to be guided by your own innate intelligence (the 'wise guide within'), transforming your patterns in whatever ways are right for you. The Metamorphic Technique is not a therapy or a treatment, as it is not concerned with addressing specific symptoms or problems. There is no need for practitioners to know about your personal or medical history. The Technique is gentle, non-invasive and completely safe. It can be used on its own or alongside conventional medicine or alternative and complementary therapies. It is easy to learn and, since no special abilities or background are needed, it is accessible to everyone. Whereas people may seek medicine or therapy because they want to be healed of something, they come to the Metamorphic Technique because they want to transform their patterns. It is an empowering tool for enabling people to 'get out of their own way', let go of past limitations and move forward in their lives.

History and background

The Metamorphic Technique has its origins in the work of Robert St. John, a British naturopath and reflexologist. During the 1960s he discovered that he could bring about significant changes by applying a light touch to particular points on the feet that reflexologists call the spinal reflexes. Later, he realised that everyone has their own capacity for self-healing and that, if he allowed it to become fully active whilst practising, then his patients would be empowered to be their own healers in a truly effective way. Since permanent, far-reaching changes on a number of levels were now occurring in his patients - changes originating entirely from within the patients themselves - he developed a body of work aptly named Metamorphosis. This unique approach distinguished it from the temporary, limited changes that his previous therapeutic approaches had achieved. Gaston Saint-Pierre, who studied extensively with Robert St. John during the 1970s, saw the potential for the development of a practical tool for self-healing and the realisation of one's potential that could be easily integrated into everyday life. He therefore went on to further develop the work and created the term 'The Metamorphic Technique' to differentiate the new direction the work was now taking. The word 'technique' is defined as a way of approaching a task that perfects itself in the practice. In 1979 he set up The Metamorphic Association, which was then registered as a charity in 1984, to promote the Technique worldwide.

What is the theory behind the Metamorphic Technique?

From the traditions of Eastern medicine to the new discoveries of science, it is generally acknowledged that energy or 'life force' underlies all forms of life. This is the basis for the Metamorphic Technique. It is now widely recognised that our energy can get 'stuck' in particular patterns. Every cell that makes up our bodies and minds holds memories of our experiences - not only from our childhood but going right back through our time in the womb to the moment we were conceived. When an experience affects us strongly, the thoughts, emotions and beliefs connected to that memory can set up energy patterns in which we become 'stuck'. In a sense, they keep us stuck in the past. These energy patterns can express themselves in a variety of ways, such as physical or mental illness, emotional problems, limiting attitudes and beliefs or repeating patterns of behaviour. In fact the Metamorphic Technique sees all mental, emotional, physical and behavioural 'problems' as symptoms or expressions of energy patterns. By using a light touch to the spinal reflex points on the feet, hands and head, the Metamorphic practitioner acts as a catalyst (something that speeds up a process of change) to the person's life force. The life force, guided by the person's innate intelligence, will then bring about whatever transformations of the energy patterns are needed. This enables the person to naturally shift those patterns that no longer serve them. The energy that was 'stuck' is released, freeing them up from past influences and allowing them to let go and move forward. While the theory can initially seem quite difficult to grasp, it is not necessary to understand it to benefit.

What does a session of the Metamorphic Technique involve?

A session usually lasts for about an hour. The recipient removes their shoes and socks and may be either sitting or lying down. The practitioner uses a light touch on the spinal reflex points in the feet, hands and head. Sessions are non-diagnostic: the practitioner does not seek to address specific symptoms or problems, so there is no need to take a case history. Some people may wish to talk about it and that is fine, but it is not necessary. Metamorphic Technique practitioners work in a detached way. This does not mean that they don't care. It simply means that they do not make judgements, impose their will or seek to direct the other person's life force in any way. This creates an environment in which that person's life force is free to do whatever is needed. The person is empowered to be his or her own healer. Most people find sessions very pleasant and relaxing.

Is the Metamorphic Technique suitable for everyone?

Yes. The Metamorphic Technique is gentle, non-invasive and completely safe. As it is the person's own life force that does the healing, it cannot do any harm. It can be safely used by anyone including children, pregnant mothers and people who are dying. The Technique can be received on its own or alongside other approaches, whether conventional medicine or alternative and complementary therapies.

Can anyone learn the Metamorphic Technique?

Yes. Although the theory behind it can initially seem quite difficult to grasp, the practice is very simple to learn and use. No special abilities or background are needed to practise. It does not involve diagnosis, so no medical training is needed. Many people take short courses so they can use the Technique with family and friends. Parents are especially encouraged to learn, so they can give the Technique to their children.

Naturopathy

What is it?

Naturopathy is a complete system of natural healthcare that believes the body has the knowledge to heal itself. Symptoms are viewed as signs that the body is attempting to heal itself, and treatment addresses the underlying causes of illness, primarily unfavourable habits of lifestyle.

The term naturopath was coined by a German homeopath, John H Scheel, to denote health promotion and treatment of the whole person with natural means. Naturopathy emerged as a separate profession when a committee of Kneipp practitioners met in 1900 and decided to broaden their practices to include all available natural methods of healing.

The aim of naturopathy is to induce health by making the individual more resilient, and the immune system stronger. The first stage being to prevent the development, or further development of disease through a variety of natural health care methods. The three basic principles of naturopathy state that:

The body has a natural drive to maintain equilibrium, symptoms of disease are viewed and indications that the body is striving to heal itself.

The root cause of all disease is the accumulation of waste products and toxins, due to poor lifestyle habits.

The body contains the wisdom and power to heal itself, provided treatment serves to enhance this power.

A naturopath will often view themselves as a teacher, whose job it is to educate and support the client. The treatment involved will vary from client to client, and will also depend on the areas of expertise that the naturopath has trained in, these may include:

Physiotherapy
Therapeutic exercise
Chiropractic manipulation of joints and soft tissue
Reflexology, acupressure or massage
Acupuncture
Hydrotherapies
Biofeedback, meditation, or autogenic training
Nutrition
Herbal remedies
Homeopathic remedies

Naturopathy can be used to treat a wide variety of illnesses and complaints. However, treatment is often dictated by the patient's willingness to change or participate. As primary care provides, naturopaths also know to refer a patient to a specialist when the illness is outside their area of expertise, or better served by modern medicine.

Neuro Linguistic Programming (NLP)

An Introduction to Neuro Linguistic Programming by Peter McNab

This short article is an introduction to Neuro Linguistic Programming (or NLP as it is now commonly known). Given the demand, I will expand on some of these ideas in future articles and also discuss more of the "how to" than is possible in this short space.

NLP has been described by one of its co-founders as "an attitude of mind leaving behind it a trail of techniques".

It is usually this "trail of techniques" which people have heard of if they have heard of NLP at all. The "Fast Phobia Relief Process" that takes only twenty minutes or relieving panic attacks in ten using "Collapsing Anchors". Both of these claims are true, by the way, and in our seminars we have taught hundreds of people these two processes and much more to very great personal and professional effect.

However, it is the "attitude of mind" that interests me more and which I would like to address in this article. But first, a little history....

Although not exclusively used for therapy and personal growth, NLP started its development over twenty years ago when John Grinder, a linguistics professor and Richard Bandler, a gestalt therapist, modelled the therapeutic skills of Virginia Satir, Milton Erickson and Fritz Perls. They became particularly interested in "how" the great and the good are successful. This was an immense shift in emphasis in terms of modelling success in any field.

Even today, most "How To" books merely tell you "What To". Look at the shelves of any bookshop and you will see a proliferation of books on "How To"... relieve stress, recover from abusive relationships, give up smoking, become a millionaire. A good look between the covers reveals lots and lots of "what to do" but very seldom will you find anything written about "How To" do it. This is what I believe NLP has added to the party. And because it is not about "what to do" there is little if any ideology attached to it. And this, of course, causes some people problems.

I well remember when I was a student teacher and later a student social worker liking some parts of various sociological and psychological theories but not all. I did not feel comfortable becoming a Freudian or a Marxist of a Jungian or a Positive Constructionist. I accepted some of Skinner's assertions and recognised that they might be useful but could not accept that we have no mind. I resolved this dilemma when I discovered NLP in 1989.

At first, I felt a bit like a renegade, a robber who only took what was best from each field but also someone who had no real depth because I was so eclectic. As the years have gone by I have begun to realise that examination through exploring "structure" and "process" reveals much more interesting phenomena. This allows us to more easily dissect the "ologies" and "isms" and to extract what is useful, and to integrate it (1).

To reduce it to its simplest elements, NLP has three "legs": Outcome, Sensory Acuity and Flexibility.

Outcome

In order to achieve any change, in order to resolve any issues, we need to know what it is that we want. The people I see in one-to-one sessions and on our seminars most often start by knowing what they don't want - "I don't want to be in this relationship", "I don't want to be smoking", "I don't want to be fat", "I don't want to be in this job", "I don't want to have these panic attacks".

In 1956, George Miller asserted that we can only consciously concentrate on seven plus or minus two pieces of information at any one time. If this is true, then we can easily see that the individual above has already used up five of those pieces; add in today's shopping and a reminder to pay the rent and we have easily filled our capacity to the full. There is literally no room to even consider what we want and so all of our concentration, all of our energy, has gone on to what I don't want.

One of the most liberating things that I help people achieve is beginning to know what they want. This in itself can be a huge shift in orientation from the past and into the future. (And if we can't stay in the present, then at least it is more fun to be in the future that in some dreadful past).

Know your outcome - know what it is that you want.

"I want to be living in an environment with fresh air pumping through my lungs", "I want to be healthily slender", "I want to be in a job where I am satisfied and amply rewarded for my efforts", "I want to be calm and serene when I want to be".

Sensory Acuity

Sensory Acuity is noticing what is going on inside and outside your body. Most people are not aware of the internal bodily sensations that we call feelings, and then further dissociate from, and call emotions.

Becoming aware of the building blocks of our experiences - the pictures that we are making, the voices that we are creating, the inner sensations that we are producing - is one of the first steps that we need to take in order to change. Once we are aware of these building blocks and also that we create themselves, we can learn how to change them to ones that are more useful to us.

For example, changing that critical voice telling us that we "have to do this" or that we "must do that" is incredibly liberating. Moving that picture of being humiliated at school further away and turning it into monochrome takes a lot of the emotion our of it and allows us to take some perspective on the experience and on the emotions - perhaps it isn't the best reference experience to take into a job interview now that you are in your thirties.

Once we have a better understanding of what is going in our own internal experience we can then extend this to others. I am sure that you have all heard of the research that 93% of our communication is at a para-verbal or non-verbal level. Like me, you probably don't completely agree with these figures. However, there is a clear message here. In our culture we put too much emphasis on the content, the words that are spoken, and we are probably missing a lot of information that is there before our very eyes and ears. Practising our sensory acuity skills and calibration skills can only enhance our relationships as we communicate with one another.

Sensory acuity at these two levels gives us vital information about what is going on for us and for others at any given moment.

Flexibility

We now know what we want and we know what we are getting. The next step is to have the flexibility to do something about it. "If you always do what you've always done, you'll always get what you've always got. If what you're doing isn't working, do something else".

Bandler and Grinder went to the world experts in their field and worked out what they did. Working on the presupposition that with the same neurology as others I can do what they can do, they modelled what these people did, learned it themselves, and started teaching it to others. They discovered what external behaviours, internal thought processes, and internal emotions you would need to have to be able to replicate the desired behaviour. This is now known as The Mercedes Model, for reasons which will become obvious when we examine the diagram below.

External Behaviours
My movements, body gestures, eye movements, and breathing make up my external behaviours.

Internal Processing
We could also call this processing our internal thoughts which consist of the pictures and words

that we create internally. These can also start to create our beliefs about ourselves and about the world.

Internal Emotions

The sensations and feelings that we have we translate into emotions. These in turn we use to start to create our values. Those things that we measure the world and ourselves against.

The interesting thing about this model is that whenever we change one aspect we automatically start to alter the other two.

Try a simple experiment to test this.

Sit in your chair. Lean forward and over. Bring your shoulders round. Breathe shallowly and look down. And feel really happy and energised. Difficult or what?

Shake that feeling off.

Now, sit up. Pull your shoulders back and breathe deeply. Push your arms out and look upwards. And feel depressed. Not easy?

Shake that feeling off.

That little experiment shows that all three aspects of the Mercedes Model are connected. Change one and the others change. Say more empowering things to yourself in a strong voice and you will find yourself thinking differently and walking and breathing differently.

In terms of therapeutic interventions it does not matter where we enter the system because wherever we enter there will be change at the other two levels. In term of elegance, the question becomes which intervention will have the most leverage and achieve the change more quickly.

However, to make any change at all, we need to know what it is that we want, notice what we are getting now for ourselves and in the world, and to be able to start to do, think and feel different things - Outcome, Sensory Acuity, Flexibility.

In this short space I have attempted a general introduction to NLP - some of the "what" but little of the "how". I will start to explore more of the "how" in my next article.

Norris Technique

What is the Norris Technique?

Patricia Norris has developed a technique to improving body alignment. A former classically trained dancer, she first became interested in developing the method whilst working with doctors in a convalescent hospital teaching remedial movement to physically disabled children. Ms Norris then went on to study many other methods of body alignment such as Pilates, yoga and the Alexander Technique, before developing her own method. It took her 25 years to perfect the Norris Technique, which concentrates on aligning the feet, knees, pelvis, shoulders and head.

The Norris Technique is not simply an exercise programme. It is a pre-conditioning through which all physical activity becomes body-benefiting exercise. Because some rewards are obvious immediately (neck and back pains are relieved, breathing becomes deeper and easier, release from stress is self-managed) there is from the beginning a strong incentive to whole-hearted commitment. People want to continue to use the technique by habit and reflex once it has been learned.

The technique is easy to learn, and requires no special equipment, it can also be learnt by people of all ages. Whilst focusing on standing correctly, an alignment for a balanced sitting position is also taught. The Norris Technique is generally taught in seminars with groups of no more than 20, however, some one-to-one teaching is available.

Nutritional Therapy

What is it?

Nutritional Therapy is not just about healthy eating. It is a form of complementary medicine in which a practitioner will work with a patient or client, helping their body rid itself of stressful substances, providing raw materials, and improving the assimilation of food in order to aid physical repair. In a recent survey of 300 people treated by a nutritional therapist, it was found that 85% of headache/migraine sufferers, 82% of people with digestive problems, 70% of people with hormone-related problems, 55% of chronic fatigue sufferers and 54% of people with skin problems reported a definite, lasting improvement, usually within two months(1).

How does it work?

How well we feel depends on the efficiency with which our body produces hormones, enzymes, prostaglandins, blood cells, antibodies and countless other substances. All these substances are made from food, but many people cannot assimilate their food properly, perhaps because of poor digestion or chronic irritation of the digestive system. They may also have a toxic overload - a build-up of unwanted waste substances that get in the way of efficient functioning. Food allergies or intolerances can also cause a lot of unpleasant symptoms, which may be delayed or chronic, and difficult to relate to a specific food.

People who have used a lot of antibiotics in the past can also be prone to dysbiosis. This is the excessive growth of undesirable bacteria and yeasts, including candida albicans (which you may have heard of) in the intestine. Dysbiosis irritates the digestive tract and this irritation may impair digestion and absorption of nutrients. Many undesirable bacteria and yeasts also produce toxic waste products which get absorbed into our bloodstream and make us feel tired or unwell.

Nutritional therapists aim to improve your body's efficiency by identifying and then dealing with these problems using a number of different types of diets, herbs and dietary supplements, according to individual need. An efficiently functioning body finds it easier to repair itself and heal itself, but if you have a serious illness much will depend on your body's powers of recuperation and on other factors such as stress.

What happens when you visit a Nutritional Therapist?

These days you can find many different books around on the subject of diets. Many of these have been written by people who have overcome their own problems with various types of diet. However, we are all different in our inheritance, our life experiences, our diets (past and present) and our combination of health problems. Therefore, what works for one will not necessarily work for someone else with a similar problem. It is for this reason that naturopathic practitioners see each person as an individual with their own set of circumstances. These circumstances may include features in common with people troubled by similar complaints but in addition there may be factors particular to you. It is discovering

134

these additional factors that is often the key to successful treatment.

Osteopathy

What is it?

A system of therapeutics, based on the normalising of the body and its functions on the principle that health depends on the maintenance of proper relationships among the various parts of the body. According to osteopathic theory, defects in the musculo-skeletal system-the muscles, bones, and joints-influence the natural function of internal organs. To correct structural abnormalities, osteopathic therapy, or treatment with the hands or by mechanical means, is used (including massage to relax stiff muscles, stretching to help joint mobility, and manipulation and high-velocity thrust techniques which can restore easy movement to the body). Using these techniques, the osteopath will endeavours to remove the abnormalities and thus re-establish the normal functioning of the body's activities.

Osteopathic medicine holds that true health involves complete physical, mental, and social well-being, rather than merely the absence of disease. The body is viewed as having a capacity for health that the osteopath can help the individual fulfil. He or she must therefore treat the whole patient, considering such factors as nutrition and mental habits in addition to the physical symptoms.

The fundamental principles of osteopathic medicine were formulated in 1874 by the American doctor Andrew Taylor Still. Still organised the first osteopathic medical school at Kirksville, Missouri, in 1892. According to Still, all diseases are caused by obstruction of arteries or nerves because of the pressure of maladjusted bones, especially of the vertebrae of the spinal column. He therefore maintained that most ailments can be prevented or cured by techniques of spinal manipulation.

Osteopaths are generally consulted to treat problems of the musculo-skeletal structure such as back pain, and many doctors refer patients to them for such treatments. It can also be used to ease pain during pregnancy, for asthma, constipation and premenstrual syndrome.

According to a Which? Way to health survey published in October 1993, an estimated 100'000 people in Britain visit an osteopath every week.

Pilates

What is it?

Pilates was developed during the 1st World War by Dr Joseph Pilates - he was a German interned by the British who used his time to teach his fellow internees exercise techniques that could be done with limited space and props, yet would aid recovery for injuries and ill health. After the war he emigrated to New York where, along with his wife Clara, he opened an exercise studio and began to promote his method. The studio was soon attracting the cream of New York's ballet and dance circles, who found the Pilates technique invaluable for rehabilitation after injury, as well as a useful addition to their own skills.

The central philosophy of the method is to strengthen the core postural muscles and develop balanced alignment through the use of slow, controlled movements and breathing. It has eight major principles: Centering, Alignment, Co-ordination, Concentration, Relaxation, Breathing, Stamina and Flowing Movements.

In recent years, with the growth of mind/body awareness, Pilates has grown and now attracts people from many walks of life - sportsmen and women, celebrities and the general public. A variety of videos are available, however it is generally recommended that beginners should initially attend a class in order to learn correct alignment before commencing with home exercise. Pilates can be taught on a one-to-one basis, or in small classes of between 8 and 12 - this ensures that the teacher is able to focus on individual needs.

The benefits to the body of Pilates have been well researched, and it is often recommended by the medical profession for chronic backache and RSI injuries. Many teachers of the discipline are former dancers with a good working knowledge of muscles and injuries, or physiotherapists who see it as a way to empower people with the means to help themselves recover from injury or pain.

Polarity Therapy

What is it?

Polarity Therapy was developed by an Austrian osteopath, chiropractor and naturopath, Randolf Stone and is another therapy that embraces both Oriental philosophies and Western therapies. He studied Ayurveda and acupuncture with particular interest in the flow of the 'life force' in the body and combined this knowledge with his Western training, to develop the basic theory of Polarity Therapy that health depends on the uninterrupted flow of energy in the body between two polar opposites.

Stone's theory of energy flow is based on the whole body as a vibrational energy field, with the spinal column as the central and neutral aspect of the body, the head and the right side of the body representing the positive electrical pole, and the feet and the left side of the body representing the negative electrical pole. The theory is similar to the Yin Yang theory of Traditional Chinese Medicine and the Chakra system of Ayurvedic Medicine. The clockwise flow between the positive and negative aspects of the electromagnetic field must be in balance and flow freely to maintain health. The spinal column has five neutral energy centres of ether, air, fire, water and earth and each of these areas corresponds to body functions and areas

Polarity Therapy treatment begins with a detailed consultation and case history details being taken. The client lies on a treatment couch, in underwear or light clothing and the therapist uses manipulation techniques and applies pressure to points on the body. Three levels of touch are used, light, medium and deep, to stimulate the neutral, positive and negative fields. Many Polarity Therapists are also qualified in counselling, as clients may be encouraged to talk through any emotional problems they are experiencing, which may be one of the reasons affecting the energy flow in the body.

Length of treatment may vary, but one session per week for around eight weeks, with occasional follow up treatments to maintain health may be suggested. Dietary advice may also be suggested as the types of food and the ability to digest may also cause blockages to the energy fields. Polarity yoga exercises may also be given to the client for home use to aid toxin removal and improve muscle tone.

Psychotherapy

The following information has been supplied by Microsoft Encarta
What is it?

Psychotherapy, treatment of psychological distress with techniques that rely heavily on verbal and emotional communication and other symbolic behaviour.

Psychotherapy differs in two ways from the informal help one person gives another. First, it is conducted by a psychotherapist who is specially trained and licensed or otherwise culturally sanctioned. Second, psychotherapy is guided by theories about the sources of distress and the methods needed to alleviate it. Because communication is the primary means of healing in most forms of psychotherapy, the relationship between the therapist and patient, or client, is much more important than in other medical treatments. The therapist's personality influences the patient and may be used quite deliberately to achieve therapeutic ends.

Attempts to ameliorate emotional and mental disorders through psychological means date from ancient times. Throughout most of history these efforts have been grounded in religious and magical beliefs. Attempts to base psychotherapeutic practices on scientific principles date from the mid-18th century, when the Austrian doctor Franz Anton Mesmer used a form of suggestion called animal magnetism. Neuroses were treated in the 19th century with such physical agents as water or painful electrical currents, both of which also depended for effectiveness on the use of suggestion. Hypnotism as a method of suggestion for alleviating certain psychological disturbances reached its height late in the 19th century, as practised by the French neurologist Jean Martin Charcot at the Salpêtrière Hospital in Paris.

Psychoanalytic Psychotherapy

Stimulated by Charcot's demonstrations of the therapeutic value of hypnosis, the Austrian doctor and founder of psychoanalysis, Sigmund Freud, used the hypnotic state, not for the purpose of suggestion, but to uncover painful and forgotten memories in his neurotic patients. By this technique, he not only attempted to help his patients but also collected the data from which he formulated psychoanalytic theory. Freud believed that during the course of a person's development unacceptable sexual and aggressive drives are forced out of consciousness. These repressed urges, constantly striving for release, are sometimes expressed as symptoms of neurosis.

Freud thought that such symptoms could be eliminated by bringing the repressed fantasies and emotions into consciousness. He first used hypnosis as the means of gaining access to the unconscious. He soon abandoned the technique, however, in favour of free association, a method in which patients were asked to report whatever thoughts came to their minds about dreams, fantasies, and memories. By interpreting these associations Freud helped his patients gain the insight into their unconscious that he believed to be curative.

Later he placed great value on what could be learned from so-called transference, that is, the patient's emotional response to therapists, which in Freud's view reflected earlier feelings towards the patient's family members. Free association and transference reactions are still central features of Freudian psychoanalysis sessions, which can take place from three to five times a week.

Divergent Psychoanalytic Schools

Some of Freud's most gifted followers disagreed with him on important aspects of theory and therapeutic technique and subsequently founded schools of their own.

Jung

Perhaps the most influential was Carl Gustav Jung, a Swiss psychiatrist, who believed that Freud overemphasized sexual instincts as a source of behaviour. Jung thought that nonsexual potentials within the person must be realized, or neuroses will develop. Jungian therapists attempt to help patients recognize their own inner resources for growth and for dealing with conflict. They see patients frequently at first, then weekly for a period of months or years. Techniques for solving immediate problems are varied and pragmatic. Dreams and art are used to draw out the patient's associations to the unconscious images that Jung believed are shared by all.

Adler

Another of Freud's students to break with him was the Austrian psychologist Alfred Adler, who also minimized the importance of instinctual sexual drives in behaviour. He believed that the smallness and helplessness of children produce feelings of inferiority in them. In reaction to these feelings, many people strive for superiority. Countering this search for power and significance is the quality of what he called social interest, that is, empathy and identification with other people. According to Adler, psychological disorders result from a faulty way of living, including mistaken opinions and goals and underdeveloped social interest. The therapist's job is to reeducate patients-to convince them of their errors and to encourage them to develop more social interest.

Fromm, Horney, and Erikson

Several of Freud's followers elaborated theories of neuroses that emphasized the role of social and cultural influences in the formation of personality. These so-called neo-Freudians include Erich Fromm,

Karen Horney, and Erik Erikson. All three emigrated from Germany to the United States in the 1930s.

Fromm believed that the fundamental problem confronted by everyone is a sense of isolation deriving from the individual's separateness. The goal of life and of therapy, according to Fromm, is to orient oneself, establish roots, and find security by uniting with other people while remaining a separate individual.

Horney believed that neurotic behaviour blocks a person's inherent capacity for healthy growth and change. The job of therapy, in her view, is to disillusion the patient of such defence blockages, that is, to identify and clarify them, and then to help the patient mobilize innate constructive forces for change.

Erikson, like Horney, was convinced that human beings are capable of growth throughout their lives. Guiding such change is the person's ego, which can develop in a healthy way when given the right environment. Failing that, a person can acquire through therapy the basic trust and confidence needed for a healthy ego. Unlike traditional psychoanalysts, Erikson, who began practice as a child analyst, usually worked with a patient's family while treating the patient.

Humanistic Psychotherapy

Begun as reaction against psychoanalytic psychotherapy, humanistic therapies are based on views of human nature that emphasize the human potential for goodness.

Carl Rogers

The oldest of the humanistic therapies is the client-centred psychotherapy of Carl Rogers, an American psychologist. Rogers believed that people, like other living organisms, are driven by an innate tendency to maintain and enhance themselves, which in turn moves them towards growth, maturity, and life enrichment. Within each person, Rogers believed, is the capacity for self-understanding and constructive change. In therapy this capacity can be realized with the help of a therapist who has certain essential qualities.

Rogers attached more importance to the therapist's attitudes than to their technical training or skills. He used the word client instead of patient to indicate that the treatment is neither manipulative nor medically prescriptive. Accurate and sensitive understanding of the client's experiences and feelings is paramount, because it helps the client focus on the experience of the moment. A second important quality in a therapist is unconditional positive regard, that is, a nonjudgemental caring for the patient. Genuineness, or an absence of sham, is a third quality that Rogers felt was essential in a therapist.

Rogers described the treatment process itself as the client's reciprocation of the therapist's attitudes. Because the therapist listens, the client learns to listen to ever more frightening thoughts and feelings until he or she reaches a stage of self-acceptance where change and growth are possible.

Gestalt Therapy

Another humanist approach, Gestalt therapy, was developed by Frederick S. (Fritz) Perls, a German-born former psychoanalyst. Perls believed that modern civilization inevitably produces neurosis, because it forces people to repress natural desires and consequently frustrates an inherent human tendency to adjust biologically and psychologically to the environment. Neurotic anxiety results; in order for a person to be cured, unmet needs must be brought back to awareness. Disavowing the psychoanalytic tradition, Perls believed that intellectual insight is powerless to change people. Instead he devised exercises designed to enhance the person's awareness of his or her emotions, physical state, and repressed needs, as well as physical and psychological stimuli in the environment. Gestalt therapy is conducted with both individuals and groups, typically in once-a-week sessions lasting up to two years.

Behaviour Therapy

In contrast to most other forms of psychological therapy, behaviour therapy is not based on a theory of neurosis. Rather, it is the application of the methods of experimental psychology to the problems of an individual who comes for treatment. Behaviour therapists, who are usually psychologists, are not directly concerned with underlying psychological forces. Instead they focus on the behaviour that is causing distress for their clients. They believe that behaviour of all kinds, normal and maladaptive, is learned according to specifiable principles. These principles have been studied extensively-in Russia, for example, by Ivan Pavlov, and in the United States by B. F. Skinner. Behaviour therapists believe that these same learning principles can be used to correct troublesome behaviour.

Regardless of the specific technique they later use, behaviour therapists begin treatment by finding out as much as they can about the client's problem and the circumstances surrounding it. They do not infer causes or look for hidden meanings; rather, they concentrate on observable and measurable phenomena. On the basis of this behavioural analysis, they formulate hypotheses about the circumstances creating and maintaining the problem. They then set out to alter the circumstances, one by one, and observe whether the client's behaviour changes as a result.

Desensitization

Of the many techniques used by behaviour therapists, one of the oldest and most common is systematic desensitization, a procedure developed by the South African psychiatrist Joseph Wolpe. Used for treating symptoms caused by excessive anxiety, this method calls for helping the client to relax and then, gradually, to approach the situations or objects that are feared.

Cognitive Approaches

Recently, behaviour therapists have begun to give more attention to the influence of thought on behaviour, spurred by such thinkers as the American psychologist Albert Bandura. Cognitive behaviour therapy uses the behavioural approach to change beliefs and habits of thought that appear to be the source of the client's distress.

Similar cognitive approaches have been devised by therapists who were trained in psychoanalysis but who become disenchanted with its theories and techniques. The oldest is the rational-emotive therapy of the American psychologist Albert Ellis, who believes that irrational beliefs and illogical thinking are the cause of emotional disturbances. In his treatment he confronts patients with their irrationality and encourages them to work vigilantly at replacing it with more reasonable thoughts and emotions.

A related technique, which has shown promise in the treatment of depression, was developed by the American psychologist Aaron T. Beck. He believes that depressed people tend to have negative conceptions of themselves, to interpret their experiences negatively, and to view the future with hopelessness. He sees these tendencies as basically a problem of faulty thinking. His treatment techniques, like strictly behaviourist approaches, are aimed at correcting the problem directly rather than understanding its possible origins in the past.

Group Therapy

Because it requires fewer therapists, group psychotherapy is less expensive than individual therapy. It may offer other advantages as well, such as demonstrating to patients that their problems are not unique. In group treatment, interactions among group members are considered the main source of change and cure; the therapist's job is to encourage and control these interactions.

Origins

Group therapy originated in Europe and the United States in the early part of the 20th century. In Europe group psychotherapy was first used by Jacob L. Moreno, a psychiatrist who had his patients act out their problems as a means of heightening their awareness of them. Moreno's "psychodrama" spread to other parts of the world and it is used for treating both neurotic and psychotic patients and also for training mental health professionals.

Many forms of group psychotherapy are practised today, and most of the theoretical orientations found in individual psychotherapy are also represented in group work. In addition, group therapy is conducted at the psychological growth centres that are part of the human potential movement. Many therapists see their patients both individually and in groups.

Family Therapy

One special type of group treatment is family therapy. Adler had worked with whole families in the 1930s, but not until the early 1950s did therapists begin treating families instead of individuals. They and their successors work from the rationale that current family relationships profoundly affect, and are affected by, an individual family member's psychological problems. Rather than explore the inner conflicts of individuals, family therapists try to promote interactions among family members, thereby enhancing the well-being of each.

New Approaches to Psychotherapy

In the late 1960s and the 1970s, a large number of new psychotherapeutic methods were devised and promoted. Many, like the earlier humanistic therapies, were born out of dissatisfaction with psychoanalytically oriented psychotherapy, which was considered too costly, too time consuming, and élitist. Some critics also believed that psychoanalytic practices were too intellectualized and rational, overly preoccupied with the past, and unnecessarily committed to preserving the Western values of individualism, achievement, and productivity. In reaction, they developed methods that emphasize emotion over reason and the present over the past and future. Others who became dissatisfied with psychoanalysis, such as Ellis and Beck, turned in a different direction and placed even more emphasis on the power of reason to overcome emotional disturbance.

Among controversial methods to have attracted public interest are primal therapy, which was devised by the American psychologist Arthur Janov, and transactional analysis, based on the work of Eric Berne. In primal therapy, patients are encouraged to relive early experiences with an intensity of feeling that had been suppressed at the time. Janov believes that such cathartic reactions free the patient from compulsively neurotic behaviour. Transactional analysis is based on the theory that a person, when interacting with others, functions as either parent, adult, or child. In therapy, usually conducted in groups, patients are taught to recognize when they are assuming one of these roles and to understand when being an authoritarian parent or an impulsive child is appropriate and to act as an adult as much of the time as possible.

Brief Psychotherapy and Crisis Intervention

Another recent trend in psychotherapy is the use of brief methods, often to help people deal with crises. These brief psychotherapies were developed partly as a result of dissatisfaction with the length of psychoanalytic therapies, which sometimes continue for many years, and partly in light of a growing understanding of the human response to crises. At critical times in life, such as after the death of a loved one, people are more susceptible to change, for better or worse. Intervening at these times not only can help them overcome the crises but may also help them to become stronger psychologically than they were before the crises.

Two major types of brief psychotherapy are practised. One type, directed at suppressing anxiety, uses supportive techniques such as reassurance, suggestion, manipulation of the environment, and medications. The other type, which uses techniques that provoke anxiety, is directed at disrupting a patient's usual neurotic defences so that change can occur. Psychoanalysis is itself an example of such an anxiety-provoking technique; as conducted by Freud, psychoanalysis was much shorter (less than a year) than is usual today.

Child Psychotherapy

Psychotherapy with children is guided by the same frames of reference used in adult psychotherapy, with the important difference that child therapists must constantly keep in mind the developmental stage of their patients. Techniques also differ. What talk is to adult therapy, play is to child therapy. Whether the therapist's orientation is psychoanalytic or behaviourist or focuses on the family as a system, the actual technique used is likely to involve play with clay, dolls, and other toys. The use of play as a means of communicating with a child in therapy was first developed by the psychoanalysts Anna Freud and Melanie Klein.

The Therapist

Psychotherapists come principally from the fields of medicine, psychology, social work, and psychiatric nursing. Their training is remarkably different, considering that their actual clinical practice may be quite similar.

Psychiatrists are doctors. In many countries, they attend medical school for a number of years, then complete a period of clinical training. They are then trained in psychiatry during a residency period lasting around three years. Psychoanalysts undergo further training of three years or more at a psychoanalytic institute. They are also required to undergo a personal analysis themselves.

Psychologists usually earn a Ph.D. degree in clinical psychology and undergo a year of supervised therapeutic practice before they are considered fully trained. Social workers specialize in mental health and earn master's or doctoral degrees before practising. Some psychologists and social workers, like psychoanalysts, take further training in an institute devoted to a particular psychotherapeutic school, and many undergo therapy as well. Psychiatric nurses usually hold master's degrees and practise primarily in hospitals.

Evaluation

The various types of psychotherapy have different goals, ranging from the psychoanalyst's ambition to alter basic personality structure and deal with existential dilemmas-problems of existence-to the behaviour therapist's more practical contention that the job of therapy is to relieve distressing symptoms. For that reason, each method of treatment must be judged against its own goal.

It is easier to measure whether a symptom has disappeared than it is to measure more far-reaching psychotherapeutic goals. Not surprisingly, behaviour therapy and other more directive, limited types of therapy are supported by evidence that is considered more scientifically valid than that used to defend psychoanalysis and related methods.

One trend has been to move away from the case histories that were once used as testimonials for a particular method and to judge treatments instead by criteria that would be applied to the evaluation of a new drug. Typically, large samples of patients receiving a standardized version of a treatment are compared with other patients who receive another treatment or no therapy at all. The goal of these investigations is to pinpoint which type of treatment is best suited for a given type of patient. This degree of specificity has so far eluded researchers, with one exception: behaviour therapy seems most effective in the treatment of phobias.

Microsoft® Encarta®.
Copyright © 1996 Microsoft Corporation.

Qi Gong

What is it?

Qigong is an Oriental therapy that combines gentle exercises with breathing techniques, meditation and visualisation to improve the circulation of Qi (life energy) in the body. It is suitable for all age groups and is particularly suited for elderly people who wish to maintain flexibility and fitness.

Qigong is based on similar principles to other Oriental health systems, in that it emphasises the need for harmony between Yin and Yang and the free flow of Qi in the meridians. Qi is believed to be the energy of the universe, and everything is made of Qi. Qi can be divided into two types - Yin and Yang. These represent two polar opposites or states of being and they are in a constant state of change. The body and mind needs a balance between the Yin and Yang aspects and an imbalance of either can lead to illness. Similarly, an imbalance between a person's Qi and the Qi of the environment they are in can also create disharmony.

The simple techniques used in Qigong help to improve the flow of Qi and therefore maintain or restore physical and mental health to optimum levels.

Qigong is usually taught and practised in a class, although once the techniques have been learned, they can be used daily as a self-help measure. Slow, flowing, rhythmical movements are used to stimulate the flow of Qi from one area to another. Awareness of ones body and how it feels, together with a focus on the breath whilst doing the exercises are an important aspect of Qigong and it is believed to help to increase vitality and promote self-healing.

Radionics

As some people claim this to be a valid form of healing, we have included it for your information.
What is it?

Radionics is said to be a form of absent healing that was pioneered in the early 20th Century by an American neurologist called Dr Albert Adams. Adams' theory was that diseased tissue would radiate an abnormal waveform - and it was by analysing this waveform that diagnosis could be made, and suitable treatment recommended.

A consultation with a Radionics Practitioner can take place over the phone or by questionnaire; a sample of blood or hair (known as a witness) is also required. Radionics practitioners claim to be able to tap into the vibrational frequencies of the patient by placing the witness on a specially designed "black box". The box is tuned to various frequency settings, and is said to be able to detect and diagnose imbalances.

Upon analysis of the results from the box, the practitioner will recommend the treatment required. This treatment could be mechanical (chiropractor), dietary (food intolerance) or be in the forms of homeopathy, herbs or nutritional supplements.

Radionics is illegal in the USA.

Reflexology

What is it?

Reflexology is a form of complementary medicine and involves a method of treatment using massage to reflex areas found in the feet and the hands. Most commonly, the feet are used as the areas to be treated.

It is said to have originated in China some 5000 years ago, when pressure therapy where used to correct energy fields in the body. It was not until around 1913 that the therapy was introduced to the west by an American ear, nose and throat consultant, Dr William Fitzgerald.

In the feet, there are reflex areas corresponding to all the parts of the body and these areas are arranged in such a way as to form a map of the body in the feet with the right foot corresponding to the right side of the body and the left foot to the left side of the body. Thus, it becomes possible to treat the whole body and the treat the body as a whole. This latter point is an important factor of a natural therapy and allows not only symptoms to be treated but also their causes.

It is thought that illness occurs when 'energy channels' in the body are blocked, causing damage to one area of another. Massage is aimed at destroying these blocks, allowing energy to flow freely again and so to heal the damage.

Reflexology does not claim to be a "cure all", but numerous different disorders seem to be responding well to this natural therapy. These disorders include such things as migraine, sinus problems, hormonal imbalances, breathing difficulties, digestive problems, circulatory problems, back problems, tension and stress.

What can you expect?

When first visiting a reflexologist, a detailed medical history will be taken. The "patient" will then be seated in a reclining chair and asked to remove shoes and socks.

The practitioner will initially examine the feet before commencing with the precise massage movement. The particular type of massage involved require the application of a firm pressure using the side and end of the thumb. In some instances, the fingers may also be employed.

All areas on both feet will be massaged. Areas corresponding to parts of the body which are out of balance will feel uncomfortable or tender when massaged and the degree of tenderness will indicate the degree of imbalance. The sensitivity of the feet varies from person to person and the trained practitioner will understand the correct pressure to apply and how to interpret the tenderness felt. The massage should not be uncomfortable, even to the most sensitive feet.

The full treatment can last up to an hour and at the end of the session, the feet should feel warm and the patient relaxed. The number of treatment sessions required will vary depending on the condition being treated.

Following treatment, it is sometime possible that the eliminating systems of the body become more active in order to rid the body of unwanted toxic matter. For example, treatment of a congested sinus may result in a cold; and constipation treatment can cause increased bowel movements. however, if treatment is correctly applied, these reactions should not be severe.

Reiki Healing
What is it?

Reiki is a Japanese word meaning Universal Life (Rei) Energy (Ki). It is a spiritual healing discipline and has its roots in ancient Buddhist teachings. The founder of Reiki, Dr Mikao Usui, spent many years seeking the knowledge of healing and found information on Reiki in Sanskrit texts. He received information on Reiki through a vision when meditating on a Japanese mountain.

Reiki is the vital life energy which flows through all living things and which can be activated for the purpose of healing. Reiki practitioners believe that everyone has the ability to connect to their own healing energy and use it for the purposes of strengthening the Ki (or life energy) of others. The Reiki therapist channels the Ki through his or her hands to the recipient, activating the body's natural ability to heal itself. When a person's Ki is strong and flowing freely, the body and mind are in a positive state of health. However, the vital energy may become weak or blocked, and this may lead to symptoms on a physical or emotional level.

A Reiki practitioner will have received 'attunements' to open their healing channels. The guidelines for the practise of Reiki are concerned with ethics and behaviour and include living in harmony with others, taking responsibility for one's own health and happiness, helping others, and being positive about all things.

Rolfing

What is it?

Rolfing is a series of deep massage treatments, which aim to re-establish the natural alignment and structural integration of the body. Dr Ida Rolf developed the system during the mid 20th century. Dr Rolf had a PhD in Biochemistry and Physiology from Columbia University; she subsequently worked at the Rockefeller Institute in Chemotherapy and Organic Chemistry. Her search for solutions to family health problems led her to study the effect of the body's structure on its functioning, hence Rolfing, or Structural Integration, was born.

Dr Rolf believed that "an effective human being is a whole that is greater than the sum of its parts". Successful, meaningful integration depends on appropriate relationships in space among the components of the body. She believed that form and function are a unity - two sides of the same coin. In order to enhance function, appropriate form must exist or be created - a joyous radiance of health is attained only as the body conforms to its inherent pattern.

What to Expect

As with Hellerwork, the client will attend a number of sessions (10), with each session building on the work of the previous. The treatments are progressive with each one concentrating on a certain area of the body; the aim is to bring harmony and alignment to the body through the loosening and balancing of the connective tissues - both the surface and deeper levels. Once a course is completed, the client can return for occasional 'treatments' to keep the structure in line.

Seichem

Seichem/Seichim/Sekhem - What is it?

This system of healing was introduced in the early 1980's, by an American called Patrick Zeigler. Zeigler had experience in the field of energetic healing which he further developed after a visit to the pyramids - the system became Seichim. Students of Zeigler have since gone on to develop the system further and it can be found under the headings of Seichem, Sekhem and SKHM. The aim of all forms is to connect with an energetic Source, and to then use this energy to promote physical, mental, emotional and spiritual healing. A Seichim practitioner's aim is to heal and help a client to stimulate their own personal development to reach a true purpose.

Seiki

What is it?

The Origins of Seiki

Seiki was developed by Akinobu Kishi, a Japanese Shiatsu Master. He was taught by his father, completing his studies with the likes of Namikoshi and Masunaga. Aged 29, Kishi became ill - Shiatsu wasn't enough, so he developed his own method of healing called Seiki - big changes occurred.

The literal translation of Seiki is 'treatment of life energy.' Originating in Shinto, inspired at times by Daoist, Zen and other great teaching traditions, Kishi's method encompasses all of this and more, looking always beyond to the very roots of our own condition.

Seiki Soho - Treatment

Seiki Soho means guidance/empathy. Everyday pressures can often manifest themselves into physical and emotional problems, distortions of life energy, indicating the body's innate willingness to seek balance. Through trusting the body it shows us how to regain balance. By using guidance and sensitivity of touch, this can be achieved.

Internal resonance (life energy or Ki) can be felt and enhanced by following a pattern of movement within the body, allowing space and time to release stagnant energy, bringing with it the potential to attain a deep sense of health and well-being. The movement we feel is the healing that we need.

The practitioner doesn't 'treat' the client, he only acts as a 'mirror' so the client can recognise how to heal 'self.'
Seiki - A Summary

Discipline and commitment are needed to become our 'real selves.' Only through continuous awareness and clearing can we develop the sensitivity necessary to feel the movement behind a physical discomfort, behind a pain or emotion, in order to release the full creative and joyful potential of our original personality and power.

Seiki has a unique approach to life and healing. It has to be experienced to be understood. It brings forth a reawakening of trust, the space to let go, the realisation that our problems are our chance, the opportunity to accept every situation as it comes (flexibility).

Seiki is a very pure method of healing self, without any compromises.

Seiki is all about 'being in the moment' - treating the whole being, with no expectations.

Seiki is performed through clothing, at floor level.

Because Seiki works from the inside out, to a certain extent, it can help all types of ailments. At times, the level of an ailment will reflect what is experienced, during and/or after a treatment. But if 'basic trust' is applied, Seiki can be the easiest, simplest thing in the world - with it comes great insight.

Shiatsu

What is it?

Shiatsu is a traditional Japanese healing art. It has its roots in ancient Oriental medicine and has evolved from Traditional Chinese Medicine and Anma, a traditional Japanese form of massage. The philosophy underlying Shiatsu is that vital energy (Qi in Chinese, Ki in Japanese) flows throughout the body in a series of channels called meridians. For many different reasons, Ki can stop flowing freely and this then produces a symptom. Shiatsu can be beneficial for a wide range of conditions - from specific injuries to more general symptoms of poor health.

Shiatsu uses touch to affect the flow of Ki in the meridians. A Shiatsu practitioner will consider your state of health, the symptoms you are experiencing and depending on your constitution and general energy levels, will use a variety of techniques to improve your energy flow. These may include gentle holding, pressing with palms, thumbs, fingers, elbows, knees and feet on the meridians, and when appropriate, more dynamic rotations and stretches. As the quality of the Ki changes, the symptoms associated with an imbalance in the movement of Ki will gradually improve. Shiatsu is a therapy that works on the individual as a complete being - the physical body and also on an emotional and/or mental level.

Each treatment will last approximately one hour. The first session will be longer since a detailed case history will be taken to develop a complete picture of your health according to the principles of Oriental Medicine. Each session usually takes place on a padded mat or futon at floor level. The client stays fully clothed.

There are several different styles of Shiatsu, and most Shiatsu Schools teach more than one style to their students. As a result, many practitioners use a blend of treatment approaches to their practice of Shiatsu. A few of the main styles are:

Namikoshi Shiatsu: (also known as shiatsu massage) places more emphasis on physical techniques developed from Anma; using pressing and rubbing to specific areas of the body to assist healing. It draws on Western knowledge of anatomy, physiology and pathology and advice on diet, exercise and lifestyle is usually given. This style tends to downplay the significance of Yin and Yang, Ki and the Meridian System.

Zen Shiatsu: Developed from Namikoshi Shiatsu by Shizuto Masunaga, this style is probably the most popular form of Shiatsu. It blends Anma with the traditional Chinese medicine concepts of Yin and Yang, Ki and Meridian theory and uses these methods to affect the flow of Ki to restore balance to the body. Masunaga extended the traditional network of acupuncture meridians to cover the whole body and used Five Element Theory which is a further classification of the types of Ki. He also devised a method of palpating the abdomen to diagnose the quality of Ki in the meridians and a theory of energy balance known as Kyo-Jitsu. Treatment involves working the whole length of the imbalanced meridian using two hands, rather than using specific points only. Advice on diet, exercise and lifestyle advice may also be given.

Tsubo Therapy: This style was developed by Katsusuke Serizawa and concentrates on the nature of the acupoints (tsubo in Japanese). It is based on the principles of Traditional Chinese Medicine and Meridian Theory, but looks for a scientific explanation of the meridian systems. Serizawa conducted research on the acupoints to demonstrate that the electrical resistance of the skin changes over a tsubo point. Treatment involves the stimulation of tsubo by means of massage, needles, electrical devices and moxa. This style is not as widespread in the West.

Sound Therapy

What is it?

Everything in the Universe is vibrating. The chair you are sitting on, or ground you are standing on is not solid, but made up of molecules all vibrating at different frequencies depending on the materials it is made from. Molecules that are vibrating give off a frequency that can be measured or converted into cycles per second (CPS) or Hertz (Hz). The human ear can hear between 20 - 22,000 CPS (Hz), so most of the frequencies given off by the objects in the world around us are either below (too dense) or above (too fine) our range of hearing (although this doesn't mean you can't feel them.)

In the days of the first space missions, Astronauts experienced what was termed as 'space-sickness'. Professor Schumann had an idea that this may be down to the astronauts being deprived of the Earth's resonance or 'song'. He fitted an instrument in the next space rocket that emitted 7.83 Hz - the Earth's frequency, and predictably, there was no more space-sickness!

Our organs, chakras and different areas of our bodies, all sing a different note, which when blended together, produce a symphony that is as unique as a fingerprint (although there are basic standard frequencies for optimum health). In an ideal world we would all be in harmony and balance, but due to the constant bombardment of factors (stress, negative energy, pollution etc) we are often being pulled 'out of tune' with our true song, therefore resulting in dis-ease.

Sound Therapy is becoming an increasingly popular way of 're-tuning' mind, body and spirit. Sound is used to correct in-balances on all levels of being using a method known as 'sympathetic resonance and entrainment'. For example, if you took two tuning forks of the same note and held them relatively close to each other. When you struck one of the forks, the other would begin to ring - why? Because the soundwaves from the tuning fork that was struck have travelled through the air and activated the tuning fork that wasn't struck, therefore the tuning fork that wasn't struck has come into sympathetic resonance with the other fork.

Sound Therapy is used in the same way to re-train the chakras and energy systems of the body to sing the right note - often by playing the note the chakra needs. This can be done using ancient and modern instruments such as singing bowls (crystal and Tibetan/Himalayan) voice, tuning forks, gong, mantra, monochord, didgeridoo etc.

Like any complementary therapy, Sound Therapy is best used as a preventative medicine. In an ideal world, we would detect and clear our in-balances before they were able to manifest in physical illness.

However, so often this is not the case, as we often keep going until forced to take notice (the piano is so far out of tune it can no longer be played) in which case, it may take longer to clear the existing blockage. However, Sound Therapy has been used with very positive results for a wide range of illnesses such as chronic pain, depression and anxiety, cysts, hormonal problems, insomnia, food poisoning, migraine etc.

This method is by no means new - many ancient civilisations used sound as a powerful tool for healing and transformation. The best practitioners today combine both ancient and modern techniques, producing an effective healing tool that is a synergy of scientific fact, intuition and thousands of years of knowledge. When choosing a sound practitioner, as with any complementary practitioner, check that they are suitably qualified and insured before choosing to work with them.

Thai Foot Massage
What is it?

Thai Foot Massage is a massage of the lower legs and feet that involves hands on stretching and massage to "open" Sen (energy) Lines, along with the use of a stick to stimulate the reflex points on the feet which correspond to the internal organs of the body. Thai Foot Massage stimulates these points to promote general health and well-being.

A Treatment in Thai Foot Massage will usually last for one hour and the therapist may spend the last 10 minutes massaging the hands and sometimes the shoulders too.

Thailand has evolved as a centre for massage, partly due to geographical location and partly to the peoples' predisposition towards massage, with traditional techniques from India and China diverging in Thailand to give us Traditional Thai Massage and Thai Foot Massage.

Thai Foot Massage takes it's origins from China where the art has been practiced for over 5000 years, and Thai Foot Massage, as seen everywhere in Thailand today, has developed from Chinese, Japanese, and Korean foot masseuses.

Traditional Thai Massage and Thai Foot Massage compliment each other beautifully. Thai Massage balances the elements of the mind and body, while

Thai Foot Massage stimulates the internal organs, giving the receiver an holistic treatment.

The benefits of a Thai Foot Massage:

Improved circulation and toxin removal.
Stimulated lymphatic drainage and immune system boost.
Reduced stiffness and improved flexibility.
Accelerated physical healing
Stress relief
Improved sleep
Clarity of mind

Thai Yoga Massage

What is it?

Thai Yoga Massage is one of the three main branches of the ancient Thai Medical system. The founder of this system is thought to have been Jivaka Kumar Bhaccha, a doctor from North India, who was the personal physician to the Magadha King Bimbisara more than 2,500 years ago. The teachings of Jivaka Kumar Bhaccha are said to have reached Thailand from India along with Buddhism in the 2nd or 3rd century BC.

Traditional Thai Medicine is based on the concept of an energy system comprising 72,000 'sen' lines through which energy is transformed and distributed in the human body. This is similar to the system of 'nadhis' found in Ayurvedic medicine and yoga.

Thai Yoga Massage works to stimulate, open and balance the flow of energy through the sen lines to assist the body in its natural tendency towards self-healing. This is achieved through rhythmic manipulation of sen lines; mobilization of joints; passive stretches and applied Hatha Yoga asanas. In practice the massage unfolds like a continuous and rhythmic dance.

Thai Yoga Massage exemplifies the four divine states of mind described in Buddhist teachings. These are: loving kindness, compassion, vicarious joy and equanimity. Thai Yoga Massage is traditionally taught and practiced with the aim of embodying these states in action. For this reason the massage is sometimes referred to as 'meditation in movement'. During a good Thai Yoga Massage the receiver would experience this meditation as a state of clear, calm and vivified embodiment.

Thai Yoga Massage is practiced on the floor. There is no need for the use of oil. The receiver can remain lightly clothed.

The Journey

What is it?

The Journey is a gentle yet powerful guided healing process. It's far reaching effectiveness and popularity is making The Journey one of the most potent forces for positive change in the UK and elsewhere. It is releasing all kinds of limitations and producing lasting benefits in situations as diverse as schools and hospices, relationships and business ventures.

There are two main reasons for the Journey's remarkable effectiveness. The first is that it uncovers the specific memories and unresolved emotions from the past that have become bound in the physical tissues of our body and are restricting us in our current lives. These physiological blocks don't just affect our health. They can also affect other areas, such as emotions, finances, work, relationships, creativity etc.

Sometimes, the old, unresolved emotions are apparent in how we react to current circumstances. Other times, the emotions may be long-buried. In either case, to be permanently free of the block, we need to uncover the root cause of our issue, the precise memory. We also need to complete and release the emotions we have unconsciously held onto. To do those things, we have to connect directly with the unconditional love at our innermost core.

This is the second reason for The Journey's effectiveness - a simple, repeatable and surprisingly quick way for people to realize that pure, absolute love for themselves. The steps involve experiencing emotions and allowing oneself to 'drop through' to a deeper experience. If we go deep enough, we fall into the fountain of peace that we recognise as our own essence or source. This is the context in which deep healing, on all levels of our being, arises.

Resting in and as our own source, the next steps of the guided process uncover and resolve those specific memories and emotions, and release the actual cellular block at the root of an issue. This is not an abstract, mental process, involving visualisation or deduction. The Journey works at the deepest levels of both our consciousness and our physiology (children sometimes describe the organ they visit in precise detail).

Each Journey is complete in itself - fully releasing blocks which may have held us back for years. It is effective for people of all ages and all kinds of issue. It restores us to our natural way of being - healthy and fully functioning with energy flowing freely in all areas.

Further reading: 'The Journey' by Brandon Bays

Thought Field Therapy

Callahan techniques® Thought Field Therapy
What is it?

Thought Field Therapy (TFT), originated and evolved by Californian clinical psychologist Dr. Roger J. Callahan, is a unique form of meridian therapy. Now in its twenty-first year of development, TFT is best described as a natural, non-invasive, drug and chemical free system for the elimination of negative or troubled emotion.

The concept and theory of the "thought field", the framework in which the causative agents of psychological disturbance exist, was proposed by Dr. Callahan to explain the observations he was making when applying the first successful treatment procedure, a rapid and easily replicable cure for most phobias. He had been treating a patient, Mary, using conventional psychotherapeutic methods for eighteen months. Her fear of water was so overwhelming that she was forced to remain in a inner room of her house whenever it rained and could just about face bathing in a few centimetres of water. Cognitive and behavioural approaches had succeeded in getting Mary to cope with her phobia to a limited extent in that she could at least approach open water, but the intense fear remained. Mary described this as being focused on her stomach.

At that time Dr. Callahan was studying Applied Kinesiology (AK) techniques. He decided to apply pressure to a treatment point on the stomach meridian, just beneath the orbit of the eye, by finger tapping on that point. Expecting nothing from such a treatment Dr. Callahan comments,

"I was totally unprepared for what happened. As I tapped under her eye, Mary said, "It's gone, my fear of water, it's gone! I don't have those awful feelings in my stomach any more." I suggested that we go down to the swimming pool adjacent to my office to see if this was really true. I expected her to resist as usual, but in fact had to hurry to keep up with her. For the first time in her life, she bent down, put her head close to the water and began splashing it on her face."

Dr. Callahan acknowledges the originator of Applied Kinesiology, Dr. George Goodheart, for the discovery of muscle testing and therapy localisation, both being fundamental to the development of TFT from this very significant beginning. Using these AK principles, Dr. Callahan developed a causal diagnostic procedure which revealed concrete evidence of the nature of the thought field. From this, and the empirical evidence obtained from many hundreds of successful TFT treatments, the concept of "perturbations" within the thought field was established. The crucial significance of the state of psychological reversal (PR), an earlier discovery, was also determined. Unique to this paradigm, the treatment of PR

- a literal reversal of meridian polarity - doubled the success rate of treatments. Single treatment points for the resolution of many phobias and love-pain, a common and powerful trauma, were the first to be defined. These were soon followed by diagnosis of generally effective treatment sequences (algorithms) for the resolution of most psychological problems. These algorithms now form the foundation of TFT practice, with causal diagnosis at the next level.

It is interesting to note the considerable significance of causal diagnosis to psychotherapy in general and especially in the development of TFT algorithms. Prior to the development of TFT no such course of determinative action existed in the practice of psychotherapy, all diagnosis simply being the application of nomenclature to common patterns of signs and symptoms. Even more remarkable is the fact that causal diagnosis allows the identification of specific treatment sequences for their resolution. Fourteen meridian points are addressed in the practice of TFT. This means that there are over 87 billion (14!) possible treatment sequences for any individual problem. Applied at random at a rate of one sequence per minute, with each point treated only once in a sequence and with no rest in between, it would take up to 165,864 years simply to begin the treatment for that single problem. However, Dr. Callahan's diagnostic procedures allow the skilled practitioner to define the exact treatment sequence required within a few minutes.

TFT theory states that if an individual suffers distress when thinking about a problem their thought field has perturbations within it. The thought field itself is regarded as tuneable manifestation of the body's energy system which contains the non-energetic active information for the generation of equally specific emotion. A perturbation in this context is defined as the entity carrying the active information which governs the expression of negative emotion when the thought field is attuned. Removal of the perturbations (i.e. the information that governs the emotional experience) from the thought field leads to loss of the negative emotion - the individual can still explore and discuss their memory of the problem but now without the accompanying distress.

It should be noted that as discrete and non-energetic carriers of information the perturbations cannot be regarded as "imbalances", "disturbances" nor "blockages" in the meridian system. This is a popular but highly unscientific viewpoint held by those with limited understanding of the paradigm and the true nature of energy, and which is sadly an identifying feature of the many therapies derived from Callahan's original work.

Consider the experience of fear. Fear is a highly ordered and precisely orchestrated experience which occurs in exactly the same manner in all members of the same species (constriction of peripheral blood vessels, dilatation of visceral blood vessels, adrenalin release, etc.), commonly known as the fight-or-flight reaction. As those events are highly ordered and balanced in both time and space, it is foolish to contend that they arise from a disordered, unbalanced or blocked system. However, the situation in which that fear response is generated may be abnormal - as is the case with a phobia (a fear of something harmless) - but the individual is still having a normal response to something which they see as a threat to their well-being, no matter how it seems to a non-phobic observer. Indeed, the perturbations associated with fear have a vital and functional purpose directly related to the survival response of the individual but which may be deactivated as a consequence of maturation. It is often a failure of this maturation process that gives rise to inappropriate emotional experience. For example, all children develop a fear of heights as soon as they begin to crawl but with maturation this fear is rapidly subsumed so that it is lost by adulthood. If this subsumption does not occur then the fear of heights remains.

Thought Field Therapy Treatment

A typical TFT algorithm treatment is conducted as follows:

The client is asked to think about their problem, thereby evoking any accompanying distress or discomfort.

They are then asked to score that emotion on a 10 or 11 point Subjective Units of Distress (SUD) scale. 1 or 0 on these scales respectively is defined as the total absence of distress, with 10 as the maximum. Children are asked to point to a position on a SUD chart or indicate the dimensions of their distress with their hands, in the same way as a fisherman would indicate the size of a fish.

The client is then asked to use two or three fingers to tap firmly, five to ten times, on specific meridian points as defined in the appropriate TFT algorithm or diagnosed sequence. For example, these might be under the eye, just below the collarbone, the back of the hand, etc.

At this point the client is asked to evoke and score their distress once more. In an uncomplicated treatment a client who reported a SUD of 10 to begin with will now report a 7.

A sequence known as the 9-gamut is then applied. The client taps a meridian point on the back of the hand continuously whilst a series of nine actions, including various eye movements, are carried out.

Once again the client is asked to evoke and score their distress. Typically, the SUD will now be reported as a 4.

The specific algorithm or diagnosed sequence is then repeated.

In a successful treatment the client will now report a SUD of 1 or 0 - or, quite often, say that they can no longer think about their problem. This is, of course, impossible (as the act of trying means that they are thinking about it) and so is taken to be a SUD of 1.

Occasionally, no change in the SUD is reported at one or more stages of treatment. This is indicative of the presence of Psychological Reversal. Once the PR correction appropriate to the stage of treatment has been administered, the predicted change in the SUD then takes place.

As the reader will appreciate, to suggest that such a series of procedures will eliminate, say, a life-long phobia is verging on the outrageous. It is for this very reason that TFT fails to enjoy a significant, if any, placebo effect. The vast majority of clients do not believe that the treatment will work. When it does, the effect on the client is so profound that they are at pains to deny that it was TFT that led to the resolution of their problem and offer alternative reasons for their recovery. In addition, the treatment procedures work with infants, young children and, it has been observed, with dogs, cats and horses . It is highly unlikely that a placebo effect would be significant in such cases. Whatever the viewpoint, the effects of TFT are predictable, saltatory, replicable by anyone and take place within minutes.

Toyohari

What is It?

Toyohari is a method of acupuncture which was developed in Japan by Kodo Fukushima - a well known blind acupuncturist, who went on to found the Toyohari Association just over 40 years ago. The theory of Toyohari is rooted in the classical texts of acupuncture which are over 2000 years old, the practice however uses innovative new techniques, including the use of needles made of different metals such as silver, gold, copper and zinc. Another development of Toyohari is the technique of "contact needling", where a silver needle or probe is held over the skin without piercing it - this method is totally painless and is used not just for those who are scared of acupuncture, but for most conditions being treated. Today there are over 1000 Toyohari acupuncturists in Japan, and in recent years Stephen Birch and Junko Ida have developed a European training program.

What to expect from a treatment

A Toyohari practitioner will firstly take thorough case notes, the client will then be asked to lie on a treatment couch and the practitioner will gently palpate the abdomen and feel the pulse at the wrist. The practitioner will then set to work to address any underlying imbalances with contact needling over selected points on the body, or stroking the skin with a rounded silver Toyohari instrument called an enshin. A technique called moxibustion may also be used to apply warmth to certain points. Toyohari is not painful, but sensations of warmth or tingling may be felt as points are stimulated. The whole process is very relaxing and a sense of deep calm and well-being may arise. A session will be between half an hour to an hour.

Toyohari is often used as a method for maintaining health, however practitioners have had clinical experience of treating a wide range of illnesses - arthritis, menstrual problems, digestive problems, skin conditions, asthma, muscular-skeletal problems, and pain relief. A Toyohari practitioner will aim to address underlying imbalances as well as the presenting symptom.

Trager Work

What is it?

Trager Work, also known as the Trager Approach, is a form of bodywork and movement which utilises gentle, rhythmic movements to facilitate the release of stress patterns, either on the mental, emotional or physical levels. It's aim is to achieve integration between the body and mind process.

Milton Trager became interested in the structure and function of the body as a result of his chronic back problem throughout his childhood. He successfully cured himself and used massage techniques to treat others for a range of disorders including chronic pain and neuromuscular problems. He then trained as a physiotherapist and doctor of medicine but continued to use a hands-on approach with his clients in his medical practise in Hawaii. He gradually developed his own approach to bodywork and together with his experience of transcendental meditation, combined his hands-on techniques with a relaxed meditative state which he called 'hook-up'.

Trager believed that physical restriction and stiffness is a learned response - an unconscious mental process that becomes habitual when repeated over time. He had witnessed a dramatic change in a patient who was extremely stiff but under anaesthetic he became completely limp. As he recovered from the anaesthesia, he returned to his original rigidity.

Trager was convinced of the affects the subconscious mind has on the body and by directing new messages through touch to release the tension from muscles and tissues, a change in habitual patterns could be achieved.

A Tragerwork Treatment

A Tragerwork session usually takes between 1 - 1-1/2 hours and takes place on a padded table with the client wearing loose, light clothing. The practitioner uses gentle rocking & vibrating movements to invoke a free, light feeling in the clients body. In a meditative 'hook-up' state, the practitioner is more able to sense tension and resistance in the client's body and when areas of tension are located, the pressure is reduced to that area. The client is passive in the process and is encouraged to relax and let go physically and emotionally. Following treatment, simple exercises are given for home use (known as Mentastics) which reinforce the subconscious messages received during treatment.

Tuina

What is it?

Tuina (a Traditional Chinese Massage) is a medical method using the arms, hands, fingers, elbows and knees as tools for treating diseases and illnesses. Tuina is also used to protect health and build up body immunity, so that disease can be stopped in its beginning acting as a preventative medical measure, without any side effects. Tuina can sometimes be mistaken for acupressure.

Tuina uses techniques and manipulations to stimulate acupuncture points or other parts of the body surface so as to correct physiological imbalances of the body and achieve curative effects. The effect of Tuina is to disperse and smooth obstructions whilst checking and restraining hyperfunction. Tuina is an important part of Traditional Chinese Medicine (TCM), which also encompasses acupuncture, herbal medicine, nutrition and exercise to treat the whole body, mind and spirit.

In summary, Tuina rectifies anatomical anomalies, alters the inner energy state of the biological system and adjusts the bio-information of the body. For soft tissue injuries, Tuina relaxes muscles and tendons and promotes smooth passage of the channels. It also promotes blood circulation and removes blood stasis.

Tuina techniques and manipulations are rigorous. Patients of Tuina treatments can be seated or may be laid on a treatment couch, whichever is the most comfortable position for both patient and practitioner. Tuina treatments are usually applied on top of loose clothing, i.e. rarely on bare skin, although herbal rubs can be used in conjunction with a Tuina treatment.

Tuina has no adverse side effects, although because it can be a powerful treatment in terms of re-adjusting the functions of the body, some patients may see an increase in frequency of visits to the bathroom, or may feel the build up and release of pressure throughout the body, or may feel slightly sedated immediately after treatment or may develop slight bruising (as blocked energy gets released). A lot depends on the patient and the nature and longevity of the disease being treated. The effects of a typical Tuina treatment, if it hasn't completely cleared any obstruction, can last up to 3 -4 days.

Tuina may be applied to treat many disorders from soft tissue injuries to many other kinds of ailments such as rheumatic pain, tiredness, lack of energy and any symptoms caused by stress or emotional problems. Tuina is even used for cosmetic purposes such as weight loss and an alternative to botox! Tuina is especially good for adults, infants, sports medicine, general health care for the elderly, rehabilitation and orthopaedics, from which many other complementary therapies have evolved as 'specialist' therapies.

Tuina works on the same basic theory as other TCM techniques : "Injury or disease causes blockages in the channels of the body. Blockages cause pain."

How many times have you massaged your temples to relieve a headache, or rubbed aching parts of your body? See...you're half way to being a Tuina practitioner already!

The History and Development of Tuina Chinese Massage

In China, Tuina dates back to the remote reign of emperor Huang, during which Tuina was called Anwu. By two thousand years ago, Tuina, called Anmo then, had developed into a widely-used medical means. 'An' meaning Press and 'Mo' meaning Rub. As time went on, Anmo was used as a term for both medical and pleasurable massage. In 1949, the Chinese government officially recognised the medical benefits of the massage and renamed this aspect to Tuina. 'Tui' meaning Push and 'Na' meaning Grasp. Tuina was officially incorporated into Traditional Chinese Medicine (TCM) as a medical therapy to be used for problems where acupuncture and herbs were less effective. The term Anmo is still used today as a term for non medical massage.

Tuina is one of the earliest medical forms of mankind and can be seen in the medical history of every old nation all over the world. The behaviour of our forefathers was to rub, press, knead, pound or stamp on themselves or their fellows bodies in order to keep out cold, get rid of discomfort and treat various injuries, continually developing their practical experiences, which gradually became what is now known as a natural therapy. At around 500 AD, the first Tuina specialists appeared, just around the Tang dynasty.

Tuina was so successful, it spread around the globe. Tuina is the basis upon which many modern complementary therapies are based, such as Shiatsu, Acupressure, Baby Massage, Deep Tissue Massage, Sports Massage, Lymphatic Draining to name but a few. Chiropractic and Physiotherapy manipulations are also founded on Tuina techniques.

Today in China, every hospital has a Tuina Department. Patients queue up from 8am every morning and have a huge range of symptoms, from prolapsed discs to frozen shoulder and sciatica, to diarrhoea, high blood pressure, migraines, knee problems, tendonitis, tennis / golf elbow to sun stroke, menstrual problems, fatigue or insomnia. Even more symptoms are treated in the infantile Tuina clinic within the department. Symptoms such as diarrhoea, constipation, vomiting, enuresis, convulsions, common cold, asthma, fever, whooping cough, chicken pox to name a few. Even infantile short sightedness is treated through Tuina massage!

Yoga

What is it?

Yoga is an ancient Indian practice using physical postures to obtain a harmony of mind, body and spirit. It is not a religion, but the discipline of breathing and concentration during practice will bring tranquility and awareness to the mind. Whilst Yoga is now taking many different forms, regular practice of any may bring about benefits, which include:

> increased oxygenation of the blood
> muscle toning throughout the body
> a clearer and more relaxed mind
> improved posture
> improved circulation of blood and lymph
> regulation of bodily functions.

Yoga Terms:

asanas - postures which can be dynamic or static

Bandha - internal energy locks which hold in prana or direct it elsewhere – they are formed when muscles are contracted

chakra - there are seven chakras along the vertical midline of the body -they are powerful areas that connect mind and body together

mantra - a chanted sound used to assist meditation practices or focus the mind mudra - a hand position that allows prana to be channeled through the body, and connect with the mind

pranayama - a breathing technique to focus on prana carrying channels

samadhi - the state of bliss that yoga aims to connect with

viniyasa - a flow of asanas and pranayamas linked together to attain maximum benefit

Yoga Styles:

Astanga

A set sequence of postures that will not vary from class to class. The sequence will move through a Primary, Secondary, and then Advanced Series, the aim of which is to leave you feeling energized and balanced with an inner alertness. It is not a beginner's method as some knowledge of postures and their correct form is required.

Bikra

A form of yoga that teaches 26 postures in a set sequence in a room heated to about 38 degrees C. It is both suitable for the beginner or the advanced student as the same pattern is always followed. The aim of the class is mostly physical improvement, although internal cleansing will also take place.

Hatha

The basis of most yoga classes, Hatha has its roots in the ancient systems first documented over 2,000 years ago. Its aim is to balance you both physically and mentally and will leave you feeling both stimulated and relaxed. It is suitable for both beginners and more advanced students, and classes will vary from teacher to teacher.

Iyengar

A very thorough form of yoga that pays attention to detail,The emphasis during a class is on correct alignment. The class is very suitable for beginners as it helps to learn each asana. The concentration involved in perfecting technique also goes to help focus the mind. A class will leave you feeling stronger, longer and calmer.

Kundalini

Perhaps the most spiritual of all the yoga disciplines. Kundalini combines asanas with mudras, mantras and breathing to allow connection with the charkas.

Power Yoga

Similar to Astanga yoga, this form was developed in America recently to offer a tough cardio workout. The classes will vary from teacher to teacher as there is no set routine.

Sivananda

This form may use mantras and meditation. It is based on 12 basic hatha postures and has a strong emphasis on breathing technique. Much of a class will also be devoted to relaxation. You will be left feeling uplifted and mentally focused.

Viniyoga

A specific one-to-one form of yoga, that aims to address as individuals needs – both mental and physical.

Zero Balancing

What is it?

Zero Balancing was developed in 1973 by Dr Fritz Smith, an American doctor, osteopath and acupuncturist. In order to understand health imbalances, he studied various methods including Rolfing, yoga, meditation and Oriental philosophies and finally developed Zero Balancing in 1975. Dr Smith practises and teaches Zero Balancing throughout the world.

Zero Balancing is a touch technique that combines Eastern and Western medicine. Treatment aims to restore a smooth flow of energy throughout the body paying attention to 'foundation' joints that act as shock absorbers for the weight distribution of the body and to breathing patterns, eye movements and stomach rumbles. The treatment is aimed at balancing the deep structures of the body, the bone and skeletal system as these contain deepest currents, to help to create stronger presence of energetic fields. The improvement to the energy flow can help to improve posture, increase harmony and the body's own self-healing ability and restore balance to the body/mind functions.

The practitioner uses gentle touch via the fingers to stretch and hold the client, who remains fully clothed. Treatment usually begins with the client sitting initially, then lying on their back on a treatment table. By applying finger pressure and holding a stretch, deep tension can be released by providing a point of stillness to allow the body to relax and re-align itself, promoting a sense of wholeness and well-being. A session will usually last for 30 to 40 minutes

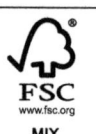